Praise for *The Vegan Athlete's Nutrition Handbook*

"As a vegan Olympian athlete, I believe that The Vegan Athlete's Nutrition Handbook *is a must-have for anyone who wants to understand how to eat plant-based for optimal nutrition, performance, and recovery. It's like having a nutrition coach by your side and will be your go-to whenever nutrition questions arise. No more confusion or feeling hungry—this book addresses ALL of your concerns, from carbohydrates and protein to vitamins and minerals to phytonutrients and recovery to how to replace your favorite foods. The fact that there are meal plans and recipes is a bonus! If you're looking for a book to help you optimize plant-based eating for athletic performance or otherwise, grab* The Vegan Athlete's Nutrition Handbook.*"*

—**Dotsie Bausch,** Olympic silver medalist and
8-time U.S. National Cycling Champion

"Plant-based eating is growing in popularity and it's no wonder people have so many questions. Is it actually healthier, and could it possibly be enough for athletes? Nichole—a registered dietitian and expert in plant-based nutrition—shows us the science and research in a digestible (zing!), easy-to-follow way, exploring the benefits along with practical applications. No matter your level of exercise or fitness, if you want to get into the details of plant-based eating and come away feeling full of info, this is your book."

—**Matt Ruscigno,** MPH, RD, co-author of
Plant-Based Sports Nutrition

T0003019

"The Vegan Athlete's Nutrition Handbook *is a guide that every plant-based athlete should have, whether they are a strength athlete or Crossfitter or an endurance athlete. Nichole has a way of turning evidenced-based nutrition and scientific information into easy-to-learn guidelines for the everyday athlete. You can relate to her personal stories as a consumer herself which makes you feel like she gets you! You will take away practical strategies to implement and of course amazing plant-based recipes to help you in the kitchen! I would absolutely recommend this for every plant-based athlete so grab yours today!"*

—**Kayla Slater,** MS, RDN, CDN, LDN, ACE-CPT
of Plant Based Performance Nutrition and Run Coaching, LLC

"Ms. Dandrea's book has been a welcome addition to my box of training tools. The Vegan Athlete's Nutrition Handbook *provides a quality resource for plant-based protein sources which is challenging to find for athletes who are plant-based or interested in transitioning to a plant based diet. Plus, the book offers information on multiple other micronutrients for athletes. The nutrition recommendations are based on multiple research studies for evidence-based advice. The recipes included are easy to prepare and delicious."*

—**Sara Love,** ND,
naturopathic physician and ultramarathoner

THE VEGAN ATHLETE'S

ATHLETE'S

NUTRITION HANDBOOK

THE ESSENTIAL GUIDE FOR PLANT-BASED PERFORMANCE

Nichole Dandrea-Russert, MS, RDN

Hatherleigh Press is committed to preserving and protecting the natural resources of the earth. Environmentally responsible and sustainable practices are embraced within the company's mission statement.

Visit us at www.hatherleighpress.com and register online for free offers, discounts, special events, and more.

THE VEGAN ATHLETE'S NUTRITION HANDBOOK

Text copyright © 2023 Nichole Dandrea-Russert

Library of Congress Cataloging-in-Publication Data is available upon request.

ISBN: 978-1-57826-904-4

All rights reserved. No part of this book may be reproduced, stored in a retrieval system, or transmitted, in any form or by any means, electronic or otherwise, without written permission from the publisher.

Cover and Interior Design by Carolyn Kasper

Printed in the United States

10 9 8 7 6 5 4 3 2 1

CONTENTS

MACRONUTRIENTS AND UNDERSTANDING HEALTH

KEY MICRONUTRIENTS

Author's Note

Hi friends! If you read my first book, *The Fiber Effect*, thank you. My intention was for *The Fiber Effect* to be like the Cliff Notes to eating fiber for optimal health. *The Vegan Athlete's Nutrition Handbook*, by contrast, might be more than you ever wished to know about plant-based eating. However, my hope is that once you have it in your library, it becomes a staple for any questions that pop up about eating plant-based for optimal health. Whether you are a weekend warrior, CrossFit enthusiast, strength-training competitor or endurance machine, this book is intended to help you incorporate more plant-based foods (or go fully plant-based) to meet your body composition, training, and recovery goals.

You will learn how many calories and how much carbohydrates and protein you need to meet those goals. You will understand why omega 3 fatty acids are so important and how to get them on a plant-based diet. You will get a deep understanding of nutrients, like protein, calcium, iron and B12, that often raise public concern around plant-based eating. Oh, and especially important, if you want to sleep really well, then jump right to the section on plant-based eating for sleep. If none of that sounds exciting to you, then simply skip to section 3 where you will find practical tips for going plant-based including resources, recipes, breakfast ideas, snack ideas and seven sample plant-based meal plans.

No matter your activity level, whether you are new to plant-based eating or have been eating plant-based for years, my intention with *The Vegan Athlete's Nutrition Handbook* is for this book to be your guide so you're fully equipped with everything you need to perform, recover and live your best through a plant-based lifestyle.

My Athlete Story

While I never really classified myself as an athlete, if" and format this new line as if we're going by the definition (to which I subscribe) that all shapes and sizes, slow speed or fast speed, elite, recreational, and everyone in between *can* be an athlete?

Then, yes. I was an athlete.

During my high school softball days, my family would cheer my "slow as a turtle" run down to first base. My hard-working legs and flailing arms made it appear as though I *might* get to the base in record time...but in actuality, despite expending a lot of energy, my speed was slow as molasses. (I was a mean slider into second base, though!)

I guess I was a decent enough player to make the college softball team at Philadelphia College of Textiles and Science (PCTS). To give you a sense of how serious we were, one of the girls had travel-size hairspray with her at all times...even in the field, hidden in her glove! During that year, I realized that softball just wasn't soul-fulfilling to me.

The combination of the mockery during my runs to first base and my can-do attitude led me to pursue running. That running turned into a huge passion in nutrition during my second year of college, so I left my design pursuits at PCTS to study nutrition at the University of Delaware.

I adored running. I lived for the runner's high, thrived on being outdoors, and discovered in myself a surprising love for races. It started with 5 and 10k's, and while I never won a race, I'd evolved a great deal since my "slow as a turtle" days—and that was enough for me! I wasn't looking to become competitive with anyone but myself. I created goals and followed running programs to help increase my speed (through sprints) and trained for a marathon—which I completed! I built up my weekly mileage over each week, did my long run on the weekend, and incorporated sprints to boost my cardio capacity.

However, even as my performance was improving, my body was suffering. I sustained injuries ranging from sciatica to Achilles tendinitis to long-run aches and pains. So, to tame my running spirit, I decided to balance it with cycling. I bought my first

Cannondale; it was (and still is) like my baby. Cycling became my thing. I loved the meditative experience of it just being me, my bike and the wide open road.

From there I moved into sprint duathlons, which was the perfect balance of cycling and running, then onto swim training for a triathlon. It wasn't easy, to say the least. I recall being on my uncle's boat with my cousins in Wildwood, NJ and in preparation for an upcoming sprint triathlon, I jumped off the boat to do a mini-training session (and probably to show off my new "swimming skills"). When I picked up my head from under the water my one cousin shouted out, "You look like a seahorse!" I couldn't disagree; the swim struggle was real and my body was straight up and down, just like a seahorse.

So I studied swimming to learn the techniques and eventually became good enough to enter my first triathlon race. During that quarter mile lake swim, the rescue boat was close by my side the whole time, and I couldn't wait to get back on land to my beloved Cannondale—but I *did* it.

With my newfound enthusiasm for triathlons came more intense training, more races...and more injuries, including not one, not two, but *three* stress fractures within a course of three months.

If you're an athlete (which I'm assuming you are, if you're reading this book), you know what an injury does to your physical and mental health. It can be devastating. All that training you do is so unforgiving when you stop. It feels like it takes months to reach a level you never thought you'd reach, than BAM! It's gone overnight and training seems to begin all over again once you're healed.

Mentally, it's rough to go from a runner's high to sitting on the sofa, waiting for your body to heal.

Then came the diagnosis. My bone scan showed osteopenia so bad that I was on the fringe—just one deviation away from osteoporosis. I was floored! For reference, prior to my injuries I'd finished my training as a dietitian and was big on low-fat dairy with each meal, along with lean meat for strength. I ate cottage cheese like it was going out of style and included chicken and potatoes or pasta with every meal.

So how was it that I, who consumed dairy with every meal and was getting well above the recommended amount of calcium, but had osteopenia at just 28 years of age (a time when my bones should be at their peak!)?

It was devastating to say the least. But this was the journey that eventually brought me to yoga. It was gentle movement that also incorporated strength building—exactly what I needed. I worked hard to get my bones to where they needed to be through yoga, strength training, and learning about the proper foods to support bone health. To my surprise, dairy didn't top the list. (In fact, I learned that countries with the highest dairy consumption also have the highest incidence of osteoporosis.)

Flash forward to now. I ditched dairy in 2013, have been eating a solid plant-based diet for years, balance running and cycling with yoga, and am now 50 years old.

And my bones look like they should have when I was 28.

So, no, I may not be the sort of athlete that typically comes to mind when you hear that word. But believe me, when it comes to supporting your body and your progress with smart nutrition through a plant-based diet? I've learned lots!

Why Vegan?

The following is my open letter to macronutrients:

Dear Macronutrients,

While I deeply appreciate all you offer, carbohydrates for energy, protein for muscle building, and fat for hormone synthesis, you seem to think you are the only nutrients that matter in training, competition, body composition and health. What you forgot to mention is that you are only one piece of the bigger picture. Your sibling, fiber, doesn't get very much attention despite its' essential role in digestion, gut health and heart disease prevention. Your cousins, micronutrients, barely get a nod despite their ability to build strong bones, boost cognition, and support hormone health. Finally, your very wise but less famous elders, phytonutrients, have been touted for their ability to reduce inflammation, support brain health, expedite recovery and improve endurance. So, why do you get all of the attention? The others may be smaller in size but just as mighty in their power to help athletes perform at their best whether it is in training, competition or life.

If there is one buzzword we see repeatedly within the athlete arena, it is macros. For those of you unfamiliar with this term, it is short for macronutrients, which include carbohydrates, protein, and fat. Many athletes, of all types, take their macros very seriously. From ensuring enough protein to carbohydrate loading to timing the perfect balance of carbohydrates and protein, athletes carefully tend to their macronutrients so that their intense hours of training do not go to waste, and they meet their body composition and health goals. It is true, macronutrients are very important!

The issue with only looking at macronutrients, is that they do not paint the entire picture. Take dairy for example. Due to its ideal balance of carbohydrates and protein, it is often recommended as a post-workout beverage because it's easy to consume during that small window for recovery nutrition (immediately following a workout) and it contains the perfect ratio of carbohydrates to protein (12 grams of carbohydrates and 8 grams of protein) for repletion. However, it is not just about carbohydrates and protein. If we look beyond building muscle, losing weight, or changing body composition and, instead, think about training goals and health, the perfect recovery drink might change.

If we create the same macronutrient composition as milk for our post-training beverage, but one that contains plant-based milk, nut or seed butter, hemp seeds, a handful of greens, banana, and berries, you get exponentially more nutrients for your macronutrient exchange. What you receive from the smoothie is almost half of your daily needs for vitamin C (collagen-building), sixty percent vitamin A (immune health), ten percent more calcium (bone health and muscle contraction), hundreds of phytonutrients (anti-inflammatory), and seven grams of fiber (gut health). (Find this recipe, Recovery Smoothie, on page 183.)

The thing is, while carbohydrates, protein and fat can be found in a variety of foods, both plant and animal-based, fiber and phytonutrients are only found in plants.* **Micronutrients are also found in a variety of foods, however, the micronutrients in animal products do not always perform equally to the micronutrients in plant products.** For example, animals have what is called heme iron. It is different from plant-based foods high in iron, such as beans and dried figs, which is called non-heme iron. Heme iron from animals is often recommended because of its high bioavailability compared to plant-based iron. While this holds true that it is more bioavailable, heme iron has also been linked to cancer and heart disease. Some experts say that it may even be the culprit in why meat increases the risk of heart disease. As it turns out, plant-based iron can be just as available as heme iron when paired with a vitamin C food. Some examples of high iron and high vitamin C combinations include beans and tomatoes (tacos!), spinach and peppers (stir fries!), and oats and berries (muffins…umm, I mean breakfast!).

Not to mention, there are elements in animal products that you will not find in plants like synthetic hormones, antibiotics and other bodily secretions that are probably better off not mentioned. Hormones are often given to animals to maximize growth quickly. These hormones are intact when we consume dairy and meat. Antibiotics are given to dairy and beef cows to prevent illness. We consume these antibiotics when we eat these products, which not only may create antibiotic resistance but may also disrupt our own microbiome.

THE VEGAN ATHLETE'S NUTRITION HANDBOOK

In addition to losing body fat and gaining muscle to give you that competitive edge, you want to feel and perform your best, right? I know you work hard in each one of your workouts or training sessions. I do not want to guess how you feel, but I am assuming that you want to bring your best to each session, perform well and not let your efforts be wasted. In addition to the short-term benefits of training, imagine an improvement in your physical performance year after year after year for the next decade.

No matter what level of athlete you envision yourself to be right now, I'll bet that you feel motivated to exercise and improve your workouts because of the health, vitality, energy and quality of life they promise to give you now and for years to come. Being an athlete goes beyond body composition. It is a lifestyle, and one that is part of optimal health and living well. The macronutrients you eat affect your sleep, mind, immune system and so much more. You are a role model for those around you, inspiring and motivating family, friends, and neighbors every time you power walk around the neighborhood, every time you cycle through your community, and every time you weight train at the gym. Sow these seeds of motivation that you work so hard to grow through feeling your best and shining your brightest.

A plant-based or plant-centered diet can help you build a healthy foundation and lay the groundwork for many factors that contribute to quality of life, and it does not have to be all or nothing. Simply eating more plant-based foods can fuel your workouts, expedite recovery, improve sleep, support immunity, create a healthy mindset and more. If these enhancements have been on your mind, if you are chasing that peak physical performance, of getting stronger every year for years to come, this is a powerful approach, and I look forward to sharing it with you.

A note about phytochemicals, also called phytonutrients: Plants are the primary source of phytochemicals because plants make them. They are chemicals or compounds produced by plants. While they are not essential to our survival, like vitamins and minerals, there are thousands of phytonutrients that are beneficial to health. Recent studies show that some phytonutrients may be present in animals who consume plants, but it's a fraction of the amount, compared to the amount in plants. Bottom line: While you may find trace amounts of phytonutrients in herbivorous animals, I wouldn't recommend eating animal products for your daily dose of phytonutrients.

MACRONUTRIENTS AND UNDERSTANDING HEALTH

CHAPTER 1

Veganism and Plant-Based Nutrition

I f you have recently shopped in a grocery store, visited a restaurant, or attended an event, you may have noticed that the options for plant-based or vegan foods are expanding. In fact, you might say that the plant-based food market is exploding. In 2021, the Plant-Based Foods Association reported that plant-based food sales increased by 6.2% percent over a record year growth in 2020 in the United States alone, bringing the total plant-based market value to 7.4 billion dollars.

These numbers reflect what consumers want: more plant-based options.

Brands are responding to the demand, but how they label their products can influence consumers' decisions to purchase them. Research shows that 58 percent of consumers would rather buy foods labeled as "plant-based" versus foods labeled as "vegan." There are negative connotations for the vegan and vegetarian terms as they are often associated with strict, bland diets that are boring. They may also be viewed as fad diets that are restrictive, difficult to follow, and diets that will leave you feeling famished after you consumed that delicious bowl of leaves and grass (this all couldn't be further from the truth when a good plant-based meal plan is in full effect).

One survey asked adults a series of questions around the terms "plant-based" and "vegan." The respondents said the term "100% plant-based" is more flexible and offers more for the consumer and describes food that tastes better and is healthier than those labeled "vegan." **Consumers see plant-based as a positive dietary choice whereas vegan is a lifestyle choice and more of a serious commitment.**

Regardless of how we label it, 52 percent of Americans are eating more plant-based foods. On a global scale, 65 percent of consumers are turning to plant-based options. The driving motivators for people to choose a plant-based diet include health, environmental, and ethical reasons. Health-related motivators to adopt a plant-based or vegan diet include food allergies and sensitivities, weight management, blood pressure control, general health benefits, and specific health conditions.

You might be wondering, what is the difference between plant-based and vegan?"

Regarding diet, plant-based and vegan terminology are often used interchangeably. However, they are not always the same. Plant-based refers to a diet that solely or mostly incorporates plant foods. It is possible that someone plant-based may also consume dairy or meat. Vegan indicates that animals are completely excluded from the diet. Those who follow a vegan lifestyle also base product choices and lifestyle decisions around animal welfare. However, vegan does not always equate to healthy foods (Oreo cookie, anyone?).

The Evolving World of Plant-Based Nutrition

In the 1980s, Dr. T. Colin Campbell, author of *The China Study*, introduced the world of nutrition science to the term "plant-based diet," using the term to define a low fat, high fiber, vegetable-based diet that focused on health and not ethics. Hence, being plant-based typically refers solely to one's diet. You may hear the terms plant-based, whole foods plant-based, or plant-forward; many people use these terms to indicate that they eat a diet that either entirely or mostly includes plant foods. Plant-forward is a style of cooking and eating that emphasizes plant-based foods but is not strictly limited to them. Meat and dairy may be included but they are usually not the main focus of the meal.

You have probably also heard of the terms vegetarian, flexitarian, pescatarian, and reducetarian.

- **Vegetarian**: a person who does not eat meat. Someone whose diet consists wholly of vegetables, fruits, grains, nuts, and sometimes eggs or dairy products.

- **Flexitarian**: One who normally eats a meatless diet, but occasionally includes meat or fish.

- **Reducetarian**: One who reduces the amount of meat they consume in order to improve their health, protect the environment, and spare farmed animals from cruelty.
- **Pescatarian**: One whose diet includes fish but no other meat.

Anyone following any of the diets above could technically call themselves a plant-based or plant-forward eater. Even the Mediterranean diet is considered plant-forward since its foundation is fruits, vegetables, nuts, beans, whole grains, and herbs. However, it also allows for fish, as well as dairy, eggs, and poultry in moderate amounts. Meat is recommended only on occasion, if at all.

Because of its recent growth in popularity, there is one last piece of terminology I would like to mention: the whole food plant-based diet. You may have heard oils are bad for you. This way of eating may avoid all oils, processed grains, and any other processed vegan foods. The "whole food" part is an important distinction since many processed vegan foods are now available in stores. For instance, a plant-based meat product like the Beyond Meat Burger may be vegan, but it would not fit in the whole food category since the pea protein in Beyond Meat is extracted from the whole pea, leaving the fiber and other nutrients behind.

The basic principles of eating whole-food, plant-based (WFPB) are as follows:

- Emphasize whole, minimally processed foods.
- Avoid animal products.
- Focus on plants, including vegetables, fruits, whole grains, legumes, seeds, and nuts.
- Exclude refined foods, like added sugars and white flour, which are processed.
- Avoid or minimize added oils.
- Pay special attention to food quality, with many proponents of WFPB promoting locally sourced and organic food whenever possible.

The Similarities Between Vegan and Plant-Based Diets

Being plant-based and vegan can go hand-in-hand. Someone may decide to be vegan for ethical reasons while eating whole plant-based foods for health. Or someone may be motivated to eat more plants for health then learn about factory farming and find themselves taking a closer look at the vegan lifestyle.

Take me as an example. I was vegan before I went plant-based. When I had the chocolate company, I partnered with animal organizations. They needed donated products for their silent auctions as a way of raising money and I had chocolate to give (well, not necessarily, but who can say no to animals in need?). During one of the silent auction events with Mercy for Animals, I watched a video of a dairy factory farm. At the time, I was mostly vegetarian, consuming dairy pretty often. It was at that moment when I realized, after watching that video, that purchasing dairy products might be contributing to more animal cruelty than eating meat. That evening, I decided to ditch dairy.

The dietitian in me needed to know if this way of eating was really healthy. Would it give me all the nutrients I need? Is it sustainable? How the heck do I even eat all plants?

The consumer in me also had questions. What will replace my daily cheese habit? What about the weekend ice cream treats, how will I live without those? And the whipped cream? Who can have ice cream without whipped cream? The struggle was real.

Transitioning to a vegan lifestyle meant some changes. From replacing the cheese with plant-based sources of calcium and protein to learning how to prepare plant-based meals that were tasty, satisfying and nourishing. The first week of plant-based eating with zero animal products involved my (unsatisfied) husband. After that first week of eating all plant-based he said, "If you don't figure out how to make something other than broccoli and pasta, you're on your own."

I honestly had no clue what I was doing when it came to preparing plant-based meals, so I invested in a few plant-based cookbooks that came with rave reviews (and mouth-watering photos). These books helped me nail down the basics of plant-based cooking. There were a handful of recipes that my husband and I both loved so they became our staples. From there, I started to experiment more. My husband even got involved! He would envision his favorite creamiest, meatiest meals and try to recreate them with plants. Honestly, I think he started having more fun in the kitchen than me. In fact, I have to admit, he is now a better plant-based cook than me!

Then there was the health aspect and advice I would give to clients. Is plant-based eating really that much better? Show me the research. What I found blew my mind. From reducing the risk of (and, in some cases, reversing) heart disease to putting diabetes in remission to reducing risk of cancer to alleviating autoimmune disease symptoms to delaying the onset of Alzheimer's disease, plant-based eating had some powerful research behind it.

In fact, here are just some benefits of eating plant-based foods:

- Reduce the risk of heart disease
- Reduce the risk of diabetes
- Lower blood pressure
- Reduce the risk of certain cancers
- Reduce the risk and slow progression of Alzheimer's disease
- Decrease inflammation
- Enhance performance
- Expedite recovery
- Increase stamina
- Support immunity
- Improve digestion
- Alleviate constipation
- Improve gut health
- Balance hormones
- Improve cognition
- Boost mood
- Improve sleep

In my current nutrition practice, I am noticing that many people do not label themselves as being plant-based or vegan but are interested in reducing their animal consumption and trying plant-based or vegan foods. The plant-based movement began with veganism, a way of living that aims to avoid animal harm for ethical reasons. It has expanded to include people who make dietary and lifestyle choices to minimize harm to the environment and their health.

The term "vegan" extends to one's lifestyle choices beyond diet alone. While these two terms are fundamentally different, they share similarities. Additionally, both are increasing in popularity and can be healthy ways of eating when planned properly.

CHAPTER 2

Calories

"Transitioning to a plant-based diet gave me the connection I needed to establish a good relationship with my body and mind. I suffered for many years from reflux and indigestion, and doctors told me I could take a pill to improve symptoms but never gave me the knowledge of the power of food as medicine. Consuming more whole plant foods and reducing animal products was my therapy to heal my aches and pains, which in turn helped me recover faster from workouts and long rounds of golf. I will never forget the time I changed my diet, it aligned with the best performance I had in my golf career (maybe coincidental), but it led me to where I am now.... pursuing a Masters in Nutrition."

—**Laura,** former professional golf player in the
Ladies European Tour Access Series

Calories are important. We could not survive without them. Our brain needs them to function. Our bodies need them to move. Our heart needs them to pump. Our lungs need them to breathe. Those are just some of the life-sustaining things that make calories essential. As you know, they can also determine our weight. If you do not eat enough calories, you lose weight and lose muscle mass. If you eat too many calories you gain weight, mostly in body fat. (I know, right? How is it fair that we lose muscle when we do not eat enough and gain fat when we eat too many?) If you eat the ideal amount supporting exactly what you need for daily functions (like breathing and thinking) plus enough to support your activity levels, from cleaning the house to working out, you maintain your weight.

It can be a bit tricky, because every single person's basic caloric needs are different based on body size, gender, genetics and more. Then when you add a variety of activity levels on top of basic needs, it can get complicated. **No two people have the same caloric needs. It is important to consider the many variables while also listening to your body's response to calories in relation to your training and health goals.**

Calories: The Basics

You may have heard "a calorie is a calorie is a calorie." **While it is true that each calorie yields the same amount of energy, foods can be metabolized and used differently, some more efficiently than others.** For example, carbohydrates, protein and fat, the macronutrients that provide calories, can each have different effects on the hormones and brain centers that control hunger and eating behavior. Macronutrients have standard amounts of calories. One gram of protein has 4 calories. One gram of carbohydrates has 4 calories. One gram of fat has 9 calories.

However, the source is important. There are many compounds in foods, besides the macronutrients, that can influence your body's process and response mechanisms. Even though each gram of carbohydrates provides four calories per gram, not all carbohydrates are created equal. For example, white bread has been refined and stripped of its fiber. Because of this, white bread may cause a spike in blood sugar, whereas whole grain bread is less processed and has its fiber intact. This allows for a slower release of sugar into the blood, meaning that while white and whole grain bread may have the same total *amount* of carbohydrates, the way they *affect* your blood sugar is very different.

Also, in general, carbohydrates digest more quickly than protein and fat, making them ideal for energy repletion during training and competitive athletic events. Carbohydrates take about 30–90 minutes to metabolize, protein can take 2–3 hours and fat takes up to 5–6 hours. If you are not training and simply want to be satiated and full after a meal then a balanced meal containing carbohydrates, protein, and fat is ideal. Think about times when you ate only a bowl of pasta or something sweet. Most likely, you were hungry shortly after you ate the meal or sweet treat.

This often results in overeating. This is very much simplified as there are many other factors that can influence hunger, including hormones and exercise, but hopefully you get the general point. Overall, the foods you eat can have a huge impact on the biological processes that control when, what and how much you eat.

Let's look at all the **nutrients** that accompany these macros. Take 100 calories of potato chips versus 100 calories of broccoli. Though technically they provide the exact same amount of energy, nutritionally, they look very different. The chips provide fat, in the form of saturated and trans fatty acids and refined carbohydrates. **These lovely little compounds can cause inflammation and damage to cells and may even contribute to the development of cancer, heart disease and many other chronic illnesses.** Chips are also devoid of essential nutrients we need to thrive, like vitamins, minerals, and fiber. Broccoli, on the other hand, provides heart-healthy unsaturated fat (a minimal amount), fiber to foster a healthy gut and enhance metabolism, and vitamin C for collagen building (important if you want pain-free joints and dewy skin) and immune function. Not only that, but it is also bursting with hundreds of phytonutrients that have been shown to fight cancer, heart disease, and other lifestyle diseases.

Let's try a better comparison when it comes to a mouthfeel and flavor substitution. When you compare a bag of potato chips to purple potatoes the same holds true. One hundred calories of a purple potato come with fiber, vitamin C, phytonutrients and more vitamins and minerals that support a healthy metabolism, anti-inflammation and optimal body functions. Try slicing potatoes super thin, tossing with a little avocado oil, salt, pepper, and garlic powder, and baking them at 400°F for 20 minutes or so, flipping halfway through. You will have yourself a crunchy "chip" you can be proud of!

When it comes to fueling your body and doing your best, a bag of potato chips may have similar macros as an air-fried purple potato. One will leave you feeling slow and sluggish and the other one will fuel you on the field from one side to the other. **It is the micro changes that create the macro results.**

How Many Calories Should You Eat in a Day?

Consuming enough calories is critical for performance, whether you are a recreational or competitive athlete. In fact, consuming enough calories is critical for overall health, both mentally and physically. Not only do calories provide fuel for a workout but eating sufficient calories also supports bone, hormone, digestive, mental, and cardiovascular health as well as prevents muscle breakdown and supports muscle growth. Just like any way of eating, getting sufficient calories on a plant-based diet is not difficult with proper planning.

Every cell in our body requires calories, or energy, to function optimally every single day. It fuels our mind and our muscles. Without it, we lose lean body mass, we begin to feel foggy, our energy starts to dip and wane. We might start to feel shaky, sweaty, and weak. For athletes, extreme incidents of calorie deficits can even result in illnesses and injuries. According to the Academy of Nutrition and Dietetics and American College of Sports Medicine Position Stands, inadequate energy intake in relation to energy expenditure can compromise performance, which in turn compromises the benefits of training. On the other hand, consuming sufficient energy will ensure adequate body composition and immune, endocrine, and musculoskeletal function and maximize training's positive effects.

Energy Needs of Athletes

The National Academy of Science, which establishes the Dietary Reference Intakes (DRIs), recommends that adults should receive 45–65% of calories from carbohydrates, 20–35% of calories from fat and 10–35% of calories from protein. Beyond the general guidelines, the amount of each macronutrient depends on the activity level. Endurance athletes' needs will be different from strength athletes' needs, which will be different from recreational athletes' needs.

The amount of calories a person needs in a day depends on metabolism at rest and activity level.

Daily energy requirements can also be influenced by specific training requirements, body composition, and thermogenesis that results from food digestion (the amount of energy it takes to digest your food). The calorie demands of training will also depend on your trained status, training distance, training duration, and environmental terrain and conditions. As you see, it can get complicated! This is why I cannot just give you a meal plan and say, "hey try this, it'll be perfect for you!" It is all so individualized.

Bear with me for a moment as we dig into lots of acronyms. **Resting energy expenditure (REE) is the energy required to maintain basic normal body functions such as keeping the lungs breathing, heart beating and brain functioning.**

These are your most basic energy needs. The thermic effect of food (TEF) is the energy needed to digest, absorb, and metabolize foods. Typically, 6–10 percent of the calories you ingest are used to metabolize food. Protein requires the most energy to digest. The energy required for basic activities (like working, grocery shopping, doing laundry) are the non-training physical activities (NTEE). The energy expenditure during training is referred to as the energy requirement for specific training or competition for an individual sport, called training energy expenditure or TEE. Once you have finished working out or a training session, your body is typically still burning excess calories. The temporary increase in REE is called excess post exercise oxygen consumption (EPOC). The total daily energy expenditure (DEE) includes the REE, NTEE, and TEE. Relative Energy Deficiency in Sport, or RED-S, is where the body is not taking in enough energy to meet demands of exercise.

The most precise way to measure caloric needs is through laboratory tests, which is not accessible to most of us. Thankfully, there are calculation methods for estimating daily energy needs. See the formulas below to determine your own caloric needs.

QUICK CALCULATION FOR ESTIMATING DAILY CALORIC NEEDS Energy Expenditure (kcal/kg/day)			
Category		**Men**	**Women**
Moderate	The activity level of a fitness enthusiast who works out for approximately 30 minutes, three to four times a week	41	37
Heavy	The activity level of an athlete who trains for 45 to 60 minutes, five to six times a week	50	44
Exceptional	The activity level of an athlete who trains one to two hours, six days a week	58	51

Data from M. Manore and J. Thompson, Sports Nutrition for Health and Performance (Champaign, IL. Human Kinetics, 2000)

If you want to be more specific, there are also formulas for figuring out your resting metabolic rate to which you can add your activity level. See the example below:

Calculating Resting Metabolic Rate

SEX	RESTING METABOLIC RATE (Mifflin-St Jeor Equation) or RESTING ENERGY EXPENDITURE
Male	10 x weight (kg) + 6.25 x height (cm) -5 x age (years) + 5
Female	10 x weight (kg) + 6.25 x height (cm) -5 x age (years) -161

CATEGORY	EXAMPLE	PHYSICAL ACTIVITY LEVEL
SEDENTARY TO LIGHT ACTIVITY	Walking or light yoga	1.2–1.375
MODERATE ACTIVITY	Fitness classes, running, cycling, weight training	1.55
VIGOROUS ACTIVITY	Endurance and elite athletes	1.7–1.9 or higher, depending on athlete

The Mifflin-St Jeor equation is predictive within 10% of calculated REE. The calculation above does not account for the potential extra 10% of calories needed by those following vegetarian or vegan diets. It also does not account for the thermic effect of food, which is 6–10% (this is not typically counted in energy calculation, it's just understood). Finally, it does not account for the excess post exercise consumption.

Once the REE is calculated, you will want to add your activity level. To simplify it, this will include basic activities plus athletic activities. There are many estimates for an athlete's physical activity level, and one individual's energy requirements can vary greatly from another. The activity level factor ranges from 1.2 for sedentary individuals to 1.9 for elite athletes.

The typical marathon runner may need to consume thousands of calories on race day to fuel a high intensity run. They may consume 2,500 calories on top of those needed to support basic metabolism. That means that some runners may need to eat 5,000 to 6,000 calories a day while an elite cyclist might consume up to 8,000 calories a day to fuel a long-distance ride. In comparison, table tennis athletes average between 3,500 to 4,200 calories per day.

Ultra-marathons are foot races that exceed the traditional marathon distance of 26.2 miles. Ultra-marathons are held all over the world, often in remote locations, on a variety of terrains, and in extremes of temperature and altitude, all of which can affect caloric needs. During these races, runners can go through a lot of physiological stress like carbohydrate depletion, dehydration, muscle damage, and oxidative stress, all of which can have both immediate and long-term health implications. These stresses can be partially addressed through eating nutritious foods. For ultra-marathon runners, the biggest nutritional challenge facing them is meeting the daily calorie demands necessary to optimize recovery and allow for prolonged and repeated training sessions. Focusing on calorically dense foods can help ultra-marathoners meet their energy needs and nutrient-dense foods to help them overcome physiological stresses. (Calorically dense foods means higher amount of calories relative to a food's weight.)

Whether you are participating in an ultra-marathon or a 5k or a 10k, running or walking, you should be proud of yourself and know that whatever movement you choose and for however long is a great thing for your body and mind. However, as noted above, the caloric needs will be dramatically different based on your activity level.

The Plant-Based Metabolism

Plant-based diets may reduce body fat through a variety of ways—more nutrient-dense foods, increased fiber intake, and less total calorie intake. Fiber can increase satiety, meaning you are satisfied more quickly and end up eating less. Increased fiber intake has also shown increased short chain fatty acid production in the gut. These short chain fatty acids have been shown to balance hormones, increase insulin sensitivity, and by doing so, improve one's metabolism.

In one cross-sectional study, researchers looked at resting energy expenditure (REE) in 26 vegetarians and 26 non-vegetarians. They found that vegetarians had a higher resting energy expenditure than non-vegetarians. The researchers speculated that it was from the vegetarian diet, lean body mass and vegetable fats consumed in place of animal fats.

Another study looked at the REE and sympathetic nervous system of 17 male vegetarians and 40 male nonvegetarians. (The sympathetic nervous system is one of two divisions of the nervous system that regulates body functions through hormones.) **Vegetarians reported more carbohydrate intake than non-vegetarians and lower fat intake.** Vegetarians were reported to have 11 percent higher resting energy expenditure. The researchers attributed this increase in energy expenditure to carbohydrate intake and its effect on the sympathetic nervous system due to an increase in norepinephrine. Norepinephrine increases heart rate and blood pumping from the heart.

In general, plant-based eaters should not need any more calories than an omnivore, but the studies above suggest that it is possible. This is good to know if you are an athlete in training, transitioning to a plant-based diet and being aware of how plant-based eating is affecting your own body and nutritional goals. If you are trying to gain or maintain weight as you transition to a plant-based diet, just be aware of the effects plant-based eating can potentially have on metabolism.

Energy Needs in Youth Athletes

Athletes who are young and still growing should pay extra attention to their calorie and nutrient needs to ensure healthy growth. Young athletes who compete in aesthetic sports (e.g., figure skaters, synchronized swimmers, gymnasts), keeping weight low over a competitive season without injury or illness or the use of extreme weight-control methods need to eat nutrient-dense foods to ensure optimal health and performance while training. What is great about a whole food plant-based meal plan is that it is naturally nutrient-dense. Calcium and iron, specific nutrients of concern in a young growing athlete, can easily be met on a plant-based diet through adequate meal planning and consuming whole plant-based foods (versus processed foods). The key is making sure that caloric needs are being met for optimal nutrition while also maintaining weight. **Meeting energy needs, while participating in high levels of exercise, is extremely important and it may be beneficial to meet with a dietitian to determine those needs and for meal and snack planning.** On the flip side, if a youth athlete is overweight, they may feel pressure to lose weight for their sport. Youth sports programs are actually an ideal time to help young athletes learn to eat for health and performance by incorporating more plant-based foods.

Energy Restriction and The Athlete Triad

Since plant-based eating is naturally lower in calories compared to meat and dairy-centric diets, athletes who are trying to lose weight may gravitate toward more plants on their plate. This is a positive thing if the purpose is to add more nutrient dense foods for overall health while trying to lose weight in a healthy way. However, if the reasoning is to restrict calories when weight loss is not warranted, this practice can be detrimental to both mental and physical health. Athletes participating in sports that emphasize leanness and aesthetics (gymnastics, diving, figure skating, distance running, cheerleading) are at increased risk for the Female Athlete Triad.

Severe energy restriction in athletes can:

- Decrease sport performance effects (due to decreased muscle strength, glycogen stores, concentration, coordination and training responses, and increased irritability).
- Increase negative health consequences (injury due to fatigue, loss of lean tissue, and poor nutrient intakes, including essential nutrients, due to limited food intake).
- Increase risk of disordered eating behaviors.
- Increase risk of dehydration.
- Increased emotional distress due to hunger, fatigue, and stress related to following an energy-restricted diet.

Female athletes who restrict energy intake long term are more likely to experience an estrogen imbalance, a halt in menses, and bone loss. This can lead to long term issues with bone health as the window for building and maintaining strong bones closes in early adulthood.

The presence of the Athlete Triad requires three things:

1. Low energy availability
2. Menstrual dysfunction
3. Bone loss

The strongest indicator of the Triad is amenorrhea, or loss of menses for three or more consecutive months. This is a result of inadequate energy to support basic needs. The body requires approximately 30 calories per kilogram of lean body mass to support normal menstrual function. Young adulthood, when you are in your 20's, is the prime bone-building window. Not receiving adequate calories to support normal menses can lead to short- and long-term bone loss.

By the way, caloric deficits can be complex and involve male athletes as well as female athletes. Relative Energy Deficiency in Sport, or RED-S refers to impaired physiological function including, but not limited to, metabolic rate, menstrual function, bone health, immunity, protein synthesis, cardiovascular health caused by relative energy deficiency. Since it can affect both male and female athletes, it is not the 'triad' (low energy, menstrual dysfunction, and bone loss) seen in females, but rather a syndrome that affects many aspects of physiological function, health and athletic performance.

As you will see in this book, consuming plant-based foods can be extremely beneficial. However, if the sole purpose is for energy restriction and it is not supporting basic physiological needs, then it is important to recognize this interruption in menses as a potential harm to skeletal structure. The loss of bone mass density is silent. It is not something you want to find out through a fracture (or multiple fractures) or later in life when a bone scan shows osteoporosis. Though the athlete triad is not always due to an eating disorder, it is a common cause. **Healthy eating should be flexible and should not cause the anxiety often seen in an eating disorder.** If you have concerns about yourself or a teammate, speak with your sports medicine physician, sports dietitian, and/or athletic trainer immediately.

Whether you are a recreational athlete who wants to lose body fat while maintaining or gaining muscle or an elite athlete trying to reach ideal body weight, working with a registered dietitian (RD), trained in sport nutrition and who understands plant-based diets, can help. It will enable you to identify and reach a realistic goal weight without the use of extreme diets or dangerous weight-loss practices or supplements.

How to Gain Weight on Plants

What appears to be a benefit for some may be a challenge for others—many people turn to plant-based eating for healthy weight loss; however, for some, whose goal is not weight loss, experience the challenge of keeping weight on when going plant-based. You *can* gain weight on a whole food plant-based diet. You just have to plan a little better than when you're consistently consuming high calorie, low nutrient, processed foods.

Foods that are considered calorically dense have a high number of calories relative to their serving size. An example includes oil. Oil is one hundred percent fat, and contains no carbohydrates or protein. Fat contains nine calories for each gram. One tablespoon of oil contains 14 grams of fat and 136 calories. Compare that to pasta, which is mostly carbohydrates (4 calories per gram) and is 110 calories per ½ cup. If you want to get even wilder, that one tablespoon of oil contains the same number of calories as 4.5 cups of broccoli. That is a lot of broccoli! However, if you drizzle that 1 tablespoon of oil over 2 cups of roasted broccoli, you will have a nutrient dense side that would provide you with additional calories. Adding it to a plate of pasta would give you even more calories. A varied plant-based diet with lots of nutrients and calories will ensure optimal health and body composition for those trying to maintain or gain.

Whole grains and starchy vegetables can also be a great caloric addition to soups, stews, stir fries and salad bowls since they are good sources of carbohydrates, which is used as the primary energy source and will prevent the body tapping into protein for energy, leading to the dreaded muscle loss. Other ideas to boost calories include: sprinkling nuts and seeds on top of oatmeal or mixing them into stir fries; blending tofu or avocado into soups and dressings; and spreading nut and seed butter over fruit or adding them to smoothies.

If you are trying to gain weight, choose your food wisely by selecting foods that pack higher calories per portion. Knowing your calorically dense foods is important for athletes who are trying to support intense training sessions, muscle growth, recovery, and optimal body composition. Try adding an additional 250–500 calories a day for weight gain.

On the next page, you'll find a table containing a variety of options for increasing your daily calorie intake for healthy weight gain.

HOW TO INCREASE CALORIES FOR WEIGHT GAIN			
Regular Meal	Higher Calorie Meal	Calories Added (approximate)	Protein Added (approximate)
Toast with plant-based butter	Toast with plant-based butter + 2 Tbsp peanut butter and 2 Tbsp chia jam	314	12
Smoothie with banana, berries, kale, plant-based milk	Smoothie with banana, kale, plant-based milk + 2 Tbsp hemp seeds and 1 avocado	338	9
Oatmeal with berries	Oatmeal with berries + 2 Tbsp flax meal and ¼ cup walnuts	251	8
Avocado toast with avocado and whole grain bread	Avocado toast with avocado and whole grain bread + ¼ cup hummus and 3 Tbsp sunflower seeds	260	10
Pasta with red sauce	Pasta with red sauce + ⅓ cup cashew cheese (for creamy red sauce)	268	12
Stir fry with rice and veggies	Stir fry with rice and veggies + 4 oz tofu and 2 Tbsp peanuts	305	21
Salad with greens, tomato, carrots, and cucumbers	Salad with greens, tomato, carrots, and cucumbers + ½ avocado, ½ cup quinoa and 2 Tbsp walnuts	307	7
Vegetable soup	Vegetable soup + 1/4 cup light coconut milk and 1 cup potatoes	201	5
Plant-based yogurt with berries	Plant-based yogurt with berries + 2 Tbsp almonds, 2 Tbsp chia seeds, 1 Tbsp hemp seeds	247	10
Banana	Banana + 2 Tbsp almond butter and 2 dates	325	7

Choosing Nutrient-Dense

Just like it is important to choose calorically dense plant-based foods when trying to gain weight, it is important to choose nutrient-dense foods for optimal health, training, competitions, recovery, focus and much more.

Nutrient-dense foods contain an abundance of vitamins and minerals, fiber, phytonutrients, protein, and unsaturated fats, but are not excessive in calories. Foods that are low nutrient density contain very little nutrients but may contain a lot of calories. These are also known as "empty calories."

For example, one slice of white bread has about 70 calories, but does not contain many vitamins, minerals, phytonutrients, or fiber. On the other hand, one slice of whole-grain bread has about the same number of calories as white bread, but four times the amount of potassium and magnesium and three times the zinc with typically 3–5 grams of fiber per slice.

Examples of nutrient-dense foods include leafy greens such as spinach, kale, and broccoli; whole grains such as oats, farro, buckwheat, quinoa, and barley; fruits such as blueberries, strawberries, and pomegranates; cruciferous vegetables such as broccoli, cauliflower, Brussels sprouts and arugula; other colorful vegetables such as tomatoes, asparagus, red onion, mushrooms and okra; and root vegetables such as sweet potatoes, purple potatoes, and carrots; and finally, legumes and legume products such as lentils, black beans, chickpeas, edamame, tofu, and tempeh.

All of these foods give you maximal nutrition for the number of calories you receive. That nutrition supports everything from metabolism to bone health to recovery to immunity. Even though nuts and seeds are calorically dense and high in fat, they are also rich in the many nutrients that plant-based foods supply. To manage weight, consider limiting nut and seed portion sizes, but still add them daily to your diet, as well as the rest of these nutrient-dense foods, to fuel your mind, your muscles, and your movement.

CHAPTER 3

Carbohydrates

"I wouldn't call myself vegan or vegetarian. I have, however, adapted many plant-based recipes into my diet, including one or two days a week consuming only plant-based foods. Overall, my digestion and 'gut health' have improved, and I love getting creative with the variety of plant-based options. My new favorites include arugula (in any form) and different types of sprouts for the crunch I crave."

—**Bobby,** recreational athlete

Carbs. The word can be a trigger. For some of you, it may trigger a visceral reaction, making you feel icky at just the thought of eating carbohydrates. For others, you may think of fuel when you think of carbohydrates since they are the primary source of quick energy to help you continue cycling and running when you feel like you're about to hit a wall. For some, just hearing the word carbohydrates makes you giddy excited. You are the person that exclaims, "Gimme all the carbs!" when someone bad mouths them.

We are about to clear the confusion around this essential macronutrient and why some shun them while others love them.

Carbohydrates: The Basics

Carbohydrates are macronutrients and one of the three ways that we receive energy through food (along with protein and fat). Each gram of carbohydrates has four calories. Macronutrients are essential for our bodies to function properly and optimally.

According to the National Institute of Health (NIH), the Recommended Daily Allowance for carbohydrates is 130 grams of carbohydrates a day, this is simply the amount your brain needs to function since your brain relies primarily on carbohydrates. However, the NIH also recommends that carbohydrate intake should be very individualized. The individualized recommendation is 45–65 percent of total calories that should come from carbohydrates. For example, a person who is consuming 2000 calories a day should include 225 (low end) to 325 (high end) grams of carbohydrates a day. That might sound like a lot, but when you break it down into smaller meals and snacks it can be very evenly distributed.

Using 250 grams of carbohydrates a day as an example, this is what it could look like:

- Breakfast: 60 grams of carbohydrates
- Lunch: 60 grams of carbohydrates
- Snack: 35 grams of carbohydrates
- Dinner: 60 grams of carbohydrates
- Snack: 35 grams of carbohydrates

Types of Carbohydrates

Carbohydrates can be classified into **sugars**, **starches**, and **fiber**. Sugars and most starches are broken down by the body into glucose (blood sugar) to be used as energy.

Carbohydrates can also be classified as **simple** or **complex**. The difference between the two forms is the chemical structure and how quickly the sugar is absorbed and digested.

Structurally, simple carbohydrates contain just one or two sugars, such as fructose (found in fruits) and galactose (found in milk products). These single sugars are called monosaccharides. Carbohydrates with two sugars—such as sucrose (table sugar), lactose (from dairy) and maltose (found in beer and some vegetables), are called disaccharides. As you can see, not all simple carbohydrates are unhealthy (beer lovers, I'm talking about fruit here). Fruit and vegetables can have simple carbohydrates as well as lots of nutrients including vitamins, minerals, phytonutrients and fiber.

You will also find simple carbohydrates in sweet sticky stuff, like candy, soda, and syrups as well as other processed foods. These types of foods are what give carbohydrates a bad name. They are made with processed and refined sugars and have zero vitamins, minerals, or fiber unless they are fortified with vitamins and minerals. Refined sugars enter the bloodstream rapidly since they are already in their simplest form, ready to be used. Plus, they do not have fiber. **Fiber helps to delay the release of sugar into the bloodstream and when a food does not contain fiber, the carbohydrates from that food is absorbed into the bloodstream more quickly.** These are the types of carbohydrates that can lead to weight gain, inflammation, fatigue, and illness. Whereas whole food, unprocessed carbohydrates help with weight management, inflammation, and long-term health.

Complex carbohydrates, also called **polysaccharides**, have three or more sugars attached to one another. They are often referred to as starchy foods and include beans, peas, lentils, nuts, potatoes, corn, and whole grains. Complex carbohydrates take longer to digest, about 60–90 minutes. The body breaks them down into smaller units of sugar that enter the bloodstream and travel to the liver. The liver converts sugar into glucose, which is carried through the bloodstream, accompanied by insulin, and converted into energy for basic body functioning and physical activity.

All carbohydrates function as relatively quick energy sources, compared to protein and fat. Simple carbohydrates can provide instant energy much more quickly than complex carbohydrates because of the rapid rate at which they are digested and absorbed. That is important during long training sessions where you need to consistently fuel with immediate energy. Simple carbohydrates can supply immediate energy to the muscles for training sessions lasting longer than 60-90 minutes.

Some of the carbohydrates we eat are stored in the liver and muscles. In cases where the glucose is not immediately needed for energy, the body can store up to 2,000 calories of it in the liver and skeletal muscles in the form of glycogen. What happens when the glycogen stores are full? Carbohydrates will be stored as fat. On the contrary, when carbohydrate intake is restricted and there is also not enough stored in the liver and muscles, the body converts protein to glucose for fuel, also known as gluconeogenesis. This is important because protein has its own important functions (as you'll see in Chapter 4), and being a backup for carbohydrates is not one of its starring roles.

Fiber is a non-digestible carbohydrate, meaning that our body does not break it down into energy. Even though we do not need it for direct energy, it is an extremely important nutrient that more than 95 percent of Americans under-consume. Fiber has been shown to help with weight management, blood sugar control, reduction of cholesterol, lower risk of colon cancer, and more. It is also essential for a healthy gut, which, if you have been paying attention to any type of media outlet that is relaying current research, you know that a healthy gut is essential to overall physical and mental health.

Fiber passes through the body whole and has traditionally been classified as **soluble** and **insoluble**. Insoluble fiber adds bulk to the stools and helps with regularity. It has also been shown to reduce the risk of colon cancer. You can find insoluble fiber in whole grains, vegetables and the seeds and skins of fruits. Soluble fiber absorbs water, helps lower cholesterol levels, and can help manage blood sugar. It slows down digestion and serves as fuel for healthy bacteria in the gut. Soluble fiber is found in oats, barley, nuts, seeds, beans, lentils, peas, and fruits and vegetables. Most foods have a combination of soluble and insoluble fiber. For example, about 25 percent of the 9.6 grams of fiber in an avocado is soluble, while 75 percent is insoluble.

The Institute of Medicine recommends that people consume 14 grams of fiber for every 1,000 calories consumed. Sources of fiber include whole plant-based foods such as fruits, vegetables, grains, legumes, nuts, and seeds. Animal products, such as eggs, meat, and dairy, do not contain any fiber.

Whole vs Processed Carbohydrates

I really do not like to classify food as "good" and "bad," however, that is how we have grown to know carbohydrates, good carbs and bad carbs, love them or hate them. Instead, I would call them what they are, whole food carbohydrates, minimally processed carbohydrates, and ultra processed carbohydrates. When you consume whole plant-based foods that are rich sources of carbohydrates you consume everything that comes with it, fiber, vitamins, minerals and phytonutrients that are beneficial for health. **When you consume ultra processed carbohydrates, you are likely getting the calories without any of the other good stuff like fiber, vitamins, minerals, and phytonutrients.** Ultra processed foods, devoid of nutrition, have also been called "empty calories." Minimally processed foods are just that—minimally processed. They often still have the fiber and some or many of the nutrients intact. Examples include whole grain bread or whole grain pasta. Even ready-to-eat fruits and vegetables, such as baby carrots, are considered minimally processed since they've been cut from their original size into their baby carrot shape.

Ultra-processed, or refined, carbohydrates are what give carbs a bad rap. These types of carbohydrates are in their simplest form. Therefore, our body digests them quickly, which can cause a rapid increase in blood sugar followed by a release in insulin, which loves to store excess carbohydrates into body fat if it is not used for energy right away. **The lack of fiber in ultra processed foods high in carbohydrates contributes further to quick entrance into the bloodstream.** They're also often accompanied by refined fat, sugar, and sodium. These are the types of carbohydrates that can lead to weight gain, inflammation, fatigue, mood swings and chronic illness.

Not only is the hormone insulin released in excess when ultra processed carbohydrates enter the bloodstream quickly, but hormones that control hunger and satisfaction, located in the lower part of the gastrointestinal tract, are not activated. This means, when ultra processed carbohydrates are digested quickly and rapidly enter the bloodstream, hunger hormones are not triggered. Therefore, your brain does not get the signal that you are full. Instead, you want more. **On the other hand, slower digesting, whole food sources of carbohydrates travel through the digestive system completely, triggering hormones that tell us we are full.** Whole, unrefined foods containing carbohydrates help with weight management, inflammation, and long-term health because of their nutrient density.

As you can see, not all carbohydrates are equal. Their structures and physiological roles can differ with some working to our benefit while others not so much.

High vs Low Glycemic Carbohydrates

The **glycemic index** (GI) is a value assigned to foods based on how slowly or how quickly the food causes an increase in blood glucose levels. Foods are ranked on a scale of 0 to 100, with pure glucose (sugar) given a value of 100. The lower a food's glycemic index, the slower blood sugar rises after eating that food. This may result in stable blood sugar, sustainable energy, and weight management. Generally speaking, refined foods often have a higher GI, and the more fiber, fat, or protein in a food or meal, the lower its GI. Foods that are low on the glycemic index (GI) scale tend to release glucose slowly and steadily, whereas foods high on the glycemic index release glucose quickly. Low GI foods have also been shown to help with weight management and diabetes. Foods high on the GI scale may help with energy repletion during long duration exercise. High GI foods can also offset hypoglycemia or insufficient blood sugar. Long-distance runners might choose high glycemic foods during a long run for instant refueling, while people with diabetes might choose low glycemic foods to avoid sharp spikes in blood sugar.

Limited studies suggest that low glycemic foods consumed before exercise could provide more sustainable energy during training, however recent studies show that it is total carbohydrates and not necessarily the type or glycemic index rating that matters. When the effects of the glycemic index have been assessed in athletes' performance, the results have been inconsistent, with evidence of improved exercise performance in some studies, but not others. One review looked at 19 studies evaluating the effect of glycemic index on performance in endurance athletes and found that there was no clear benefit of consuming a low glycemic index pre-exercise meal for endurance performance.

While the evidence does not necessarily support consuming a low glycemic index meal pre-exercise for improved performance, limited research shows that eating a low glycemic meal before exercise can sustain blood sugar levels, which, in theory, seems like it would help with long-term energy during exercise. A low GI meal might look like whole grain bread with nut or seed butter, brown rice and lentils, or slow-cooked oats with berries, plant-based milk, and nuts. High glycemic index foods include whole or mashed potatoes, white or whole wheat bread, instant oats, and watermelon. Experiment with high and low glycemic foods (during training, not competition) to see if lower glycemic index foods work for you before exercise and provide sustained energy during exercise. **Remember that every calorie counts and choosing calories that are nutrient dense are most beneficial for overall health and performance, both physically and mentally.** For example, choosing whole potatoes instead of white bread will provide you with more nutrients such as vitamin C, potassium and magnesium.

Carbohydrates and Athletic Performance

Athletes, from recreational to elite, are often searching for an edge whether it is a new technique, training regimen, supplement or nutrition program that might help to shave seconds off their personal best time, gain strength necessary to compete at a higher level, meet body composition goals, or optimize recovery. These are called ergogenic aids, substances that are used to improve any form of activity performance in humans. Among the most popular and probably the most misunderstood ergogenic aids that athletes use to enhance performance is diet. Thanks to a large amount of emerging research over the past 50 years, the link between physical performance and nutrition is now well known.

A panel of four experts met in 2017 for one day and reviewed the latest nutrition research regarding the dietary needs of serious athletes, trained-but-not-elite performers, as well as weekend warriors. They discussed issues such as the potential impact of high-quality, nutrient-dense carbohydrates versus low-quality, calorie-dense simple sugars on performance and the evolving role of protein in an athlete's diet. **The panel stated that different types of athletes, whether they are long-distance cyclists or hockey players or recreational 10-K runners, have unique nutritional needs for performance and recovery.** That said, a few constants exist— the need for carbohydrates, protein, and fluids in varying combinations (depending on the sport and the intensity of the training regimen). They also said that food should ideally come from natural, whole-food sources, to fuel the training, recovery, and adaptation requirements. Although dietary protein and fat can provide energy to perform physical activity, carbohydrates is the preferred nutrient that is most efficiently metabolized by the body and the only macronutrient that can be broken down fast enough to provide energy during periods of high-intensity exercise.

The experts also explained that there's research showing that many athletes do not consume enough carbohydrates to fully replenish muscle glycogen stores, which can lead to decreased performance, especially when strenuous exercise is performed on a regular basis. Less-than-optimal daily carbohydrate intake is likely a result of demanding training schedules, busy lives, confusion regarding the benefits of dietary carbohydrates, and a misunderstanding of how much carbohydrates is needed.

Anaerobic exercise also is fueled almost entirely by carbohydrates. If carbohydrate stores are depleted, the body switches to protein for fuel and not fat since fat requires aerobic activity to be used as fuel. During aerobic training, long term ketone (fat) use for energy has been shown to impair cognitive and physical performance in athletes. Without enough carbohydrates, glycogen stores drop significantly after both aerobic and anaerobic exercise, which could affect subsequent performance if it is not replaced. Some athletes may argue that they can function and perform fine with lower carbohydrates, but there is a difference between functioning and performing optimally.

Restoring Glycogen for Recovery and Adaptation

Aerobic performance is directly related to glycogen stores as muscle glycogen is the predominant fuel source used during endurance training. **Once glycogen is depleted, athletes become fatigued, and performance may suffer.** Carbohydrate stores in the liver and muscle can become depleted after about 90 minutes of training, which is why it is important to fuel during training sessions lasting longer than 90 minutes. What is the best type of carbohydrates to eat during training? Finding the right mix of carbohydrates for you is what is most important. Everyone is different and not one type or mix of carbohydrates is right for everyone. Research shows that fueling with either simple carbohydrates or complex carbohydrates is equally effective, one is not better than the other. Both are equally effective in restoring glycogen in the liver and muscles. It may be a banana (simple carbohydrates) or a pb & j sandwich (combo of simple and complex carbohydrates).

Immediately after exercise, consuming high glycemic carbohydrates seems to be most effective in increasing muscle glycogen stores. In one study, researchers fed participants either high- or low glycemic meals during 24 hours of recovery after completing two hours of cycling exercise at 75 percent VO2max and four 30-second, all-out sprints. The high-GI diet resulted in greater glycemic and insulin responses, followed by greater repletion of muscle glycogen.

After intense workouts, athletes are physically depleted, mentally exhausted, and may be dehydrated. Recovery nutrition is essential, having three primary goals: refuel, rehydrate, and repair and build. Replenishing vital nutrients, rehydrating, and restoring electrolyte balance, repairing damaged muscle tissue, and minimizing inflammation accomplish these goals. Including nutrient-dense carbohydrates foods can help ensure adequate consumption of nutrients vital to health, recovery, repair, adaptation, growth, and performance. Ensuring adequate recovery enables athletes to better respond to increases in training volume and intensity and perform at their best.

Refueling

After intense training, athletes need to consider when, what and how much to eat and drink. These considerations depend on the sport, the training program, environmental factors, the athlete's health history, body composition, performance goals, and physical conditioning. These three components, when, what and how much, are referred to as "nutrient timing."

The rate at which muscle glycogen is depleted depends on the intensity of physical activity. Basically, the greater the intensity, the more quickly muscle glycogen is depleted. For example, repeated sprinting can quickly lower muscle glycogen stores, even though the total time of activity might be brief (an example being, 10 × 30 second sprints with short recovery intervals). Sports that include quick sprints include basketball, hockey, and swimming. In comparison, endurance athletes who train for hours at a time will also experience a marked decline in muscle glycogen, however the depletion occurs at a slower rate than that of the sprinter. High-glycemic carbohydrates foods, such as potatoes will replenish glycogen stores when consumed immediately following workouts since muscle tissue is sponge-like and will rapidly soak up glucose from the high-glycemic carbohydrates.

Exercise sensitizes muscle tissue to certain hormones and nutrients; therefore, muscle is most responsive to nutrient intake during the first 30 minutes following training. This window of opportunity diminishes as time passes, however, certain types of exercise, such as resistance training to the point of muscular fatigue, keeps that metabolic window open for up to 48 hours.

Immediately following exercise, research shows that nutritious, carbohydrate-rich foods that are easily digested and absorbed can optimize glycogen synthesis, which is important when training multiple days in a row or more than one training session a day. When immediate glycogen synthesis is required, it is recommended that athletes consume approximately 0.5 to 0.6 gram per kg of body weight of rapidly absorbed carbohydrates every 30 minutes for two to four hours after exercise (or until the next full meal).

A simpler method is 1.5 grams of rapidly absorbed carbohydrates per kg of body weight immediately after exercise. For a 150-pound athlete (68 kg) that is 102 grams of carbohydrates (1.5 grams per kg) or 34 grams of carbohydrates every 30 minutes for two to four hours post exercise. **If the athlete delays carbohydrates consumption by two hours or more, glycogen synthesis can be reduced by 50 percent.** In addition, ingesting protein along with carbohydrates can increase muscle glycogen stores when insufficient total carbohydrates is consumed or when carbohydrate intake is consumed in intervals spread out by more than one hour.

Carbohydrates content in post-training snacks or mini-meal examples. Depending on your needs, adjust the portion size. Veggies are not included as they provide a minimal amount of carbohydrates for repletion, but they provide lots of nutrients for recovery. Feel free to add them to any or all meals and snacks. For example, adding tomato, radish, and greens to avocado toast, greens to a smoothie or carrots and celery along with the hummus and crackers.

Food	Carbohydrates Content	Calories
1 large banana + 2 Tbsp peanut butter	32 g	310
PB & J (2 slices wheat bread, 2 Tbsp peanut butter, 1 Tbsp natural preserves)	40 g	383
Smoothie (1 banana, ½ cup plant-based milk, 1 cup berries, 2 Tbsp hemp seeds)	46 g	353
Whole grain crackers and hummus (15 crackers, ½ cup hummus)	34 g	310
1 cup yogurt + ¼ cup homemade granola + ¼ cup berries	31 g	459
½ cup oatmeal, ½ cup plant-based milk, ½ cup berries + ¼ cup walnuts	30 g	405
Avocado toast (1 slice whole grain bread + ½ avocado, 1 slice pineapple)	34 g	391
Peanut butter + banana toast (2 Tbsp peanut butter, 1 sliced banana, 1 slice whole grain toast)	43 g	378
Homemade granola bar, 1 cup plant-based milk, 1 apple	34 g	307
Rice and lentil bowl (½ cup rice + ½ cup lentils)	38 g	239
Mashed potato bowl with black beans and salsa (½ cup mashed, ½ cup beans, 2 Tbsp salsa)	35 g	264
Hummus wrap (1 whole grain tortilla, ¼ cup hummus, veggies)	30 g	256
Trail mix (¼ cup nuts + ¼ cup ounce dried fruit)	30 g	293
Baked sweet potato (medium), ½ cup lentils, 1–2 Tbsp tahini-based sauce	42 g	323
Banana walnut bread (slice) + 2 Tbsp almond butter	32 g	401

Carbohydrate Loading

Your body can store about 2,000 calories of carbohydrate (the form of glycogen) in your liver and muscles. Glycogen can be broken down into glucose that can be used for fuel, but it lasts only 90 to 120 minutes of vigorous activity. To maximize glycogen stores, some athletes practice what is called carbohydrate loading (also called glycogen supercompensation). **Eating carbohydrate-rich foods before a competition or event provides athletes with the energy that they need to sustain an increased level of activity for a longer duration.** One review looked at carbohydrate loading in stop and go sports, such as soccer, basketball, field hockey and rugby, where players repeatedly have brief bouts of high-intensity exercise followed by lower intensity activity.

Energy production during brief sprints in these sports comes from intramuscular phosphocreatine (see supplementation chapter for more info on creatine!) and glycogen. Continuous periods of multiple sprints can drain muscle glycogen stores, leading to a decrease in power output and a reduction in general work rate during training and competition. Increasing liver and muscle carbohydrate stores before competition helps delay the onset of fatigue during this time. One study showed that carbohydrate intake during exercise can also improve performance and delay onset of fatigue. Finally, ingesting carbohydrate immediately after training and competition will rapidly recover liver and muscle glycogen stores.

Back in the 1960s and 1970s, athletes would deplete their glycogen stores by exercising to near exhaustion the week before competition and then eat a very low carbohydrate diet for three days. This was followed by three days of 80–90 percent of carbohydrate intake ("carbohydrate loading"). The latter three days, the carbohydrate loading phase, was effective in super-compensating glycogen stores, however the very low carbohydrate phase caused weakness, irritability, and a compromised immune system, making athletes more susceptible to infection.

Today, it is suggested that carbohydrates are 55–60 percent of energy up until three days before competition, then increasing carbohydrate intake up to 80–90 percent of energy intake. This is just making sure that carbohydrate stores are maximized before competition.

Eating a high-carbohydrate diet may help athletes perform at their best. However, eating an unusually high amount of carbohydrates right before an event could also hinder athletic performance by causing gastrointestinal distress. This is why it is important to "practice" which foods work best for you during training, not during competition or events. Foods eaten immediately before an event should be the same foods consumed during training. Nothing new on race day, a golden rule in sports nutrition, also applies to carbohydrate loading.

Carbohydrates Needs of Athletes

Consuming the ideal amount of carbohydrates depends on a variety of factors, including body size, the type of sport, the duration of training, training adaptation goals, and body composition goals. To determine how much carbohydrates you need, you can start with a basic calculation, but it will ultimately take trial and error to see what amount, type and timing works best for you. It can also vary depending on your training schedule, rest days, and competition days, if you compete.

In general, it is recommended that competitive athletes consume 6–8 grams of carbohydrates per kilogram per day during training and up to 12 grams of carbohydrates per kilogram per day during the highest intensity training. For example, a 150-pound athlete would need 409 to 545 grams of carbohydrates per day during training (6–8 grams of carbohydrates per kilogram). When not training, or low intensity training it is recommended that athletes consume 3–5 grams of carbohydrates per kilogram of body weight a day. Again, for a 150-pound athlete, it would be 204 to 340 grams of carbohydrates per day. This is also the amount that would pertain to recreational athletes. Again, it really depends on the sport, frequency of training, duration and intensity of training, and body composition goals.

Use the formula below for estimated carbohydrates needs and see what works best for you. I often suggest keeping a time journal of foods consumed and a training log to see how much carbohydrates you consumed before, during and after training, and evaluate how that amount and type of carbohydrates affects your training session, as well as your short- and long-term goals. For example, perhaps you skipped breakfast the day of a long run and noticed that the run was not your strongest. It is helpful to go back to see exactly what you ate, or did not eat, that may have impacted your run.

CARBOHYDRATE NEEDS BASED ON ACTIVITY LEVEL (INTERNATIONAL OLYMPIC COMMITTEE RECOMMENDATIONS)	
Physical Activity Level	**gm/kg of body weight per day**
Low-intensity or skill-based activity	3–5
Moderate exercise (about 1 hour a day)	5–7
Endurance program, moderate to high intensity, 1–3 hours a day	6–10
Strength-trained athletes	4–7
Extreme commitment, moderate to high intensity, >4–5 hours a day	8–12

https://www.ncbi.nlm.nih.gov/pmc/articles/PMC5753973/

D. Enette Larson-Meyer, PhD, RDN and Matt Ruscigno, MPH, RDN, authors of *Plant-Based Sports Nutrition* (a book I highly recommend), suggest that every athlete should count their carbohydrate intake at least once to learn more about which foods are the richest sources of carbohydrates and to determine which foods are best to consume before, during and after a race. They suggest counting carbohydrates for at least two days using Nutrition Facts labels and other sources (the USDA Nutrient Database is a great resource). Once you have calculated your overall carbohydrate intake, compare it to your estimated carbohydrate needs to see if you are meeting those needs and how you are feeling. If you feel like you could be stronger in your training sessions, then consider adding more carbohydrate-rich foods to meet your estimated needs. If you already feel strong and are meeting your training and body composition goals, then you are probably doing great with the current amount you are eating.

For more information on good, nutrient-dense high carbohydrate whole grains that can help fight inflammation, speed recovery, replete energy stores and so much more, see page 215 in Tables and References.

ONE LAST WORD ABOUT LOW CARB DIETS

Still unsure about "carbs?" Here are a few more tidbits of information that may change your mind about eating whole plant-based food sources of carbohydrates like whole grains, starchy vegetables, beans, peas, and lentils.

Hormone imbalance can be a result of a low carbohydrate diet. Some evidence suggests that low-carbohydrate diet can increase the stress hormone, cortisol. The hypothalamus, pituitary, and adrenal glands work together to regulate stress hormones. This is called the HPA axis. Hormones can control mood, digestion, the immune system, metabolism, and energy levels. Lack of overall calories, including carbohydrates, can create stress in the body, releasing stress hormones that can negatively affect mood, digestion, the immune system, and metabolism. Also, whole food sources of carbohydrates naturally stimulate the production of serotonin, which stabilize the mood and give feelings of well-being. Whole grains are also rich in nutrients that support mood and mental health, like B vitamins, magnesium, and zinc.

Fiber-rich carbohydrates also help to stabilize blood sugar. Not only fiber, but plant-based proteins found in many whole grains play a part in slowing the absorption of glucose (or sugar) into the blood (for example, amaranth has 5 grams of fiber and 9 grams of protein per cooked cup!). For those following a plant-based diet, whole grains can contribute a decent amount of protein.

Carbohydrates fuel the brain and nervous system. When blood glucose runs low, you can become irritable, disoriented, and lethargic, and it could be difficult to concentrate or perform simple tasks.

Sleep can also be affected by a low carbohydrate intake. (Fast-track to Chapter 18 on sleep to learn more about how carbohydrate intake can create a slumber sleep.) This is only observational, but I notice in my own practice that when people restrict carbohydrates- and fiber-rich foods throughout the day they seem to have more food cravings at night. Typically, when they fill up their day with sufficient calories, carbohydrates, protein, and fat from whole plant-based foods through satisfying meals, they make sensible snack choices at night and do not have those same cravings.

Whole, unprocessed, plant-based carbohydrates-rich foods can fuel your brain, your muscles, and your gut. Will you be a carb shunner or a carb lover?

CHAPTER 4

Protein

"'How do you get enough protein?' was my biggest hurdle to overcome until I heard several vegan world class athletes and bodybuilders on the Rich Roll podcast. I thought if they can perform at their level without eating meat or dairy, there is no reason for me to worry if I can get enough protein! So, my journey began about 3 years ago and never looked back. My daily elimination became effortless and I first noticed my facial skin started to feel so much better. Ironman and marathon trainings get intense and brutal sometimes, but I noticed I was recovering better and felt stronger for a longer duration. I literally started to feel like I was running on clean fuel. My mind and body are happier with whole food plant-based eating."

—**Izumi,** Ironman and marathon competitor

Protein is probably the number one concern when someone is transitioning to a plant-forward or plant-based diet. The most common question from those unfamiliar with a plant-based diet is "but where do you get your protein?" The concern makes sense since we have been programmed to believe that protein is only found in animal products like dairy, eggs, and meat. We also know that protein is important for bones, hormones, digestive enzymes, absorption of nutrients, rebuilding and replenishing all kinds of cells, not to mention it is the most important macronutrient for building muscle mass.

Some fad diets focus solely on protein. High protein foods on grocery shelves have additional protein added to them to make them even higher in protein. Protein powders, initially created for athletes, are now found in 46 percent of Americans' pantries. When I see clients who want to eat more plants or transition to fully plant-based, choosing a replacement protein is often their biggest challenge. Once they remove animal protein, what is left? Oftentimes, I see an empty plate. They often resort to huge salads or mounds of vegetables, which have some protein, but not enough to be satisfied or sufficient to build muscle mass or maintain other important functions. A diet of lettuce alone is just not sustainable. With thousands of edible plants in the world, there are plenty of options!

When you choose to eat plant-based protein, you are choosing to not only eat the protein, but also all of the plant compounds that come with it and have been shown to optimize health. By choosing plant-based sources of protein, you may lower your risk of heart disease, reduce blood pressure, lower risk of diabetes, reduce risk of certain cancers, optimize your workouts and training, expedite recovery, support your immune system and so much more.

There is one difference between animal protein and plant-based protein that may concern those looking to optimize their protein intake while minimizing carbohydrates: **plant protein also comes with carbohydrates**. Unless you are choosing protein powder that has been processed so that the only macronutrient you receive is protein, then you're getting carbohydrates with that protein (however, tofu and tempeh have minimal carbohydrates per serving). For example, a three-ounce portion of meat contains 21 grams of protein and zero carbohydrates while one cup of lentils contains 18 grams of protein and 24 grams of carbohydrates (this is net carbohydrates or actual carbohydrates used for energy once you subtract the fiber).

This presents a dilemma for those watching carbohydrate intake while maximizing protein intake, which circles back to the question, do we really need to minimize carbohydrate intake to meet our goals? Remember that it is the type of carbohydrates that matters. The lentils also contain 16 grams of fiber which is essential for optimizing gut health. **When gut health is optimized, metabolism is optimized.** Finding the perfect balance of carbohydrates, protein and fat is very individualized based on your age, height, weight, training regimen and body composition goals, but what is certain is the nutrients you receive from plant-based protein trump the nutrients found in animal-based protein.

What's more, studies show that swapping out animal protein with plant protein may decrease mortality in both men and women. One large study from Harvard University, looking at over 100,000 people, found that replacing animal protein with plant protein was associated with lower risk of mortality. Another study involving over 400,000 men and women showed that replacing just three percent of animal protein with plant protein decreased risk of mortality. The cause of increased mortality from animal protein may be due to many variables, including other beneficial nutrients found in plants that may be beneficial; increased levels of insulin-like growth factor 1 (IGF-1) associated with animal product consumption; a metabolite called trimethylamine N-oxide (TMAO) that increases with animal product consumption and is associated with heart disease; or the sequence of amino acids in plants versus animals. The benefits of plant protein over animal protein may also be due to less environmental pollutants found in plant protein compared to animal protein.

The natural next question is can you build muscle and optimize performance following a plant-based diet? The short answer is yes! Look at Torre Washington, Lilian Aguilar, Patrik Baboumian, and Robert Cheeke (I highly recommend you pause reading and Google them if this is the first time that you are hearing of them). They follow a plant-based diet and it is clearly working for them in both performance and body composition. However, they are not just wonders of the universe. First, they train hard. Second, they eat whole plant-based foods. There is plenty of research to back up their success that can also be applied to you! Gaining muscle, increasing strength, and optimizing performance on a plant-based diet just requires a little planning, but once you have that plan, it easily becomes a part of your lifestyle.

Protein: The Basics

Amino acids are the building blocks of proteins. There are 20 amino acids, nine of which are **essential**, meaning our body does not make them, so we need to obtain them from food. The nine amino acids that our body cannot make include histidine, isoleucine, leucine, lysine, methionine, phenylalanine, threonine, tryptophan, and valine. We have many types of proteins in our body with amino acid sequencing that makes each one different with their own unique specialty, whether it is enzymatic, transport, structure, hormones, antibodies, storage, or muscles. Proteins serve a variety of functions within cells. The functions of individual proteins are as varied as their unique amino acid sequences and structures. Amino acids can also serve as a source of energy in the absence of carbohydrates, a process called gluconeogenesis, which becomes important during training or when insufficient calories are obtained.

Protein is found in muscle, bone, skin, hair, and virtually every other body part or tissue. It makes up the enzymes that power many chemical reactions and the hemoglobin that carries oxygen in your blood. It assists with metabolism by providing structural support and acting as enzymes, carriers, or hormones. Proteins are responsible for nearly every task of cellular life, including cell shape, inner organization, waste cleanup, and routine maintenance. Bottom line, protein is pretty important!

PROTEIN TYPES AND FUNCTIONS		
Type	Example	Function
Digestive enzymes	Amylase, protease, lipase	Breaks down starches, proteins, and fats
Transport	Hemoglobin	Transports oxygen to tissues
Structural	Collagen	Provides strength, support and elasticity of tissues
Hormones	Insulin	Promotes glucose uptake in cells
Defense	Immunoglobulins	Fights foreign pathogens
Contractile	Actin, myosin	Affects muscle contraction

Protein Needs for Athletes

The National Academy of Medicine does not have a set recommendation of protein intake for athletes. However, in a 2016 joint position paper on nutrition and athletic performance, the American College of Sports Medicine (ACSM), the Academy of Nutrition and Dietetics (AND), and Dietitians of Canada recommend higher protein intakes for athletes and also suggest that athletes should give some attention to timing of protein intake. They do not differentiate between strength and endurance athletes in making the following recommendations:

- Dietary protein intake necessary to support metabolic adaptation, repair, remodeling, and for protein turnover generally ranges from 1.2 to 2.0 grams per kg day.

- Daily protein needs should be met with a meal plan providing a regular spread of moderate amounts of high-quality protein across the day and following strenuous training sessions. Muscle protein synthesis is maximized by consumption of 0.3

grams protein per kg body weight every three to five hours, including consumption of this amount within two hours following exercise.

Research indicates that protein requirements should be tailored to reflect sport-specific and training-goal requirements. Differences in training, desired outcomes, competition, and nutrition require an individualized approach and should be continuously adjusted and adapted. There is strong evidence to suggest that the timing, type, and amount of protein intake influence post-exercise recovery and adaptation.

For athletes, protein needs may increase depending on the type of activity. For example, if you are a recreational fitness enthusiast who exercises on the weekends or a few times a week, you may be good with .8–1 gram of protein per kilogram of body weight per day. This may also apply to athletes who are taking time off between training and only performing in light maintenance training during the off season. However, strength and power athletes might need more like 1.6–1.7 grams of protein per kilogram of body weight per day. The recommendations for endurance athletes are 1.2–1.4 grams of protein per kilogram of body weight per day. However, high intensity training, up to 40 hours a week, may require up to 2.0 grams of protein per kilogram of body weight per day, depending on the type of training and whether or not muscle gain is important. Athletes need more protein during training and competition based on the amino acids that are needed to promote muscle protein synthesis, repair exercise-induced muscle damage and maintain protein needs for all of the basic body functions mentioned above.

For athletes, protein also plays a role in exercise performance and exercise adaptation. **Adaptation is the body's response to a new exercise or if you load your body in a different way, it responds to training and adapts by increasing its ability to cope with that new load.** The balance between Muscle Protein Breakdown (MPB) and Muscle Protein Synthesis (MPS) is known as Net Protein Balance (NPB). Achieving a positive NPB through increased MPS promotes exercise recovery, adaptation, and muscle growth. You can achieve NPB by receiving sufficient calories and protein, as well as eating a variety of plant-based foods with quality protein.

Getting Sufficient Calories

Research shows that those who take in enough calories to support their training needs and eat a variety of whole plant-based foods get enough protein without having to calculate how much protein they need in a day. This is because protein is naturally found in so many plant-based foods and can easily be obtained from the diet as long as caloric needs are met. However, if caloric intake is restricted for either weight loss or simply not enough is consumed to support training needs, more protein will be needed to support the functions of protein listed previously.

Optimizing Protein Intake on a Plant-Based Diet

The optimization of protein intake for plant-based athletes may require some attention on the quantity and quality of protein consumed. You have probably heard of branched chain amino acids and perhaps even taken them as an individual supplement for muscle growth and repair. Three of the nine essential amino acids are branched chain amino acids (BCAA), leucine, isoleucine, and valine. Branched chain amino acids have been shown to build muscle, decrease muscle fatigue and alleviate muscle soreness. Leucine is one of the branched chain amino acids that is key in building muscle mass. Studies show that it is the most important amino acid to stimulate muscle protein synthesis. In one study, people who consumed a drink with 5.6 grams of BCAAs after their resistance workout had a 22 percent greater increase in muscle protein synthesis compared to those who consumed a placebo drink. It also plays an important role in promoting recovery and adaptation from exercise. **Leucine can also help prevent deterioration of muscle with age.** One study looked at 368 individuals 35–65 years old over a six-year period and found that leucine intake was associated with lean body mass (LBM) changes in those older than 65 years, with no effect seen in those younger than 65 years. Older participants who received the most leucine (7 grams per day) experienced LBM maintenance, whereas lower intakes were associated with LBM loss over six years. This study shows that greater leucine intake along with adequate protein intake may be associated with long-term lean body mass retention in a healthy older population.

Fun fact: the action of lifting weights stimulates leucine uptake (as well as other amino acids) by the muscles, which triggers muscular growth.

Can you get leucine in plants? **Research shows that plant proteins can maximally stimulate muscle protein synthesis and provide enough leucine when a variety of whole plant-based foods are consumed.** Getting sufficient leucine means including soy, lentils, black beans, chickpeas (and other legumes), nuts and seeds with every meal or snack. For example, instead of just eating oatmeal, add almonds and hemp seeds to the oatmeal. Instead of only eating a banana, add a nut or seed butter to the banana.

Plant-based foods with the highest amount of leucine include vital wheat gluten (seitan), seaweed, hemp seeds, peanuts, pistachios, pumpkin seeds, chia seeds, almonds, pecans, sesame seeds, cashews, oats, flax meal, Brazil nut, soybeans, buckwheat, black beans, navy beans, kidneys, chickpeas, lentils, navy beans, mung beans, and lima beans. That is a lot! Getting enough leucine should be a piece of cake. Err...I mean a piece of plant-based nutrition bar made with nuts and seeds.

OLDER POPULATIONS

Active older adults (over 65 years of age) may need more protein to build and maintain muscle for optimal health. Greater protein needs for older individuals are not yet reflected in the RDAs. However, it is clear that not only do older people progressively lose muscle as they age but they also resist building new muscle. Starting around the age of 50, muscle loss, known as sarcopenia, can range anywhere from 0.5 to 2 percent of total muscle mass each year. It used to be thought that increased protein intake in older people would lead to bone loss and kidney issues.

However, now experts believe that more protein can benefit bone health and maintain muscle mass. Research shows that adequate protein intake coupled with resistance exercise can overcome the resistance to build new muscle. Consuming up to 35 percent of daily calories as protein is safe for older adults unless there is a medical reason to restrict protein. Pair inactivity with low protein intake, and continued muscle loss with age is inevitable. A shortfall of protein may put older people at considerably high risk for conditions such as sarcopenia, osteoporosis, disabilities, falls, fractures, and illness.

Current studies suggest that most people over age 65 should consume about 1 gram to 1.2 grams of protein per kilogram of body weight per day to both gain and maintain muscle mass and function. One study showed that just 33 percent of women and 50 percent of men who were between the ages of 60–99 years met the RDA (.8 grams/kg/day) for protein. Plant-based eaters over the age of 50 can boost their protein intake by consuming soy products, such as tofu, soymilk, and soy yogurt, lentils, beans, nuts, and seeds. Spreading protein out between meals may also be helpful. Seniors should strive for 30 grams of protein at each meal and include a bit of protein in snacks as well. Breakfast can often be a neglected meal when it comes to protein. A tea and toast breakfast is not conducive to maintaining muscle health. Add a nut or seed butter to the toast and a sprinkle of hemp seeds to boost the protein in that breakfast.

Excess Protein is Not Necessarily Better

Consuming more protein than you need will not stimulate more muscle growth. Instead, the protein will be used for either energy or stored as fat. Also, some studies show that excess protein may increase urinary calcium losses, which may affect bone health. Using the chart below will help to determine your individual protein needs.

Estimating Protein Needs

Determine body weight in kg: (weight in pounds divided by 2.2)

Multiply your weight by the amount of protein needed to support your activity level.

0.8 grams protein x weight (kg) = RDA

1.2 grams protein x weight (kg) = lower range recommended for athletes

2.0 grams protein x weight (kg) = upper range recommended for athletes

Example: 150-pound strength-training athlete with a goal of building muscle may need 1.5–2.0 grams of protein per kilogram of body weight will need 102–136 grams of protein a day.

150 divided by 2.2 = 68.18 kg

68.18 x 1.5 = 102 grams of protein

68.18 x 2.0 = 136 grams of protein

Timing of Protein

The International Society of Sports Nutrition (ISSN) is a non-profit leading organization who provides science-based information and application of sports nutrition and supplement information for athletes. **They recommend that athletes, from recreational to elite, meet their daily protein needs through evenly spaced meals and snacks, i.e., eating every three hours during the day.** When looking at improving body composition, consuming 20–40 grams of high-quality protein every three to four hours appears to favorably affect muscle protein synthesis rates when compared to other dietary patterns and is associated with improved body composition and performance outcomes. Eating high quality sources of protein immediately after exercise or up to two hours after exercise can also stimulate muscle protein synthesis.

What does 20–40 grams of plant-based protein look like?

Snack or Meal	Protein Content (grams)	Leucine Content (grams)
Peanut butter (2 Tbsp), hemp seed (2 Tbsp) and jelly on whole grain bread (2 slices)	24	.9
Hummus (½ cup) and buckwheat crackers (20)	23	.6
Quinoa (1 cup) bowl with chickpeas (1 cup) and broccoli	23	1.5
Homemade granola (1 cup) with soy milk (1 cup) and extra almonds (1 ounce)	26	1.9
Buckwheat chia pancakes (four 4") with almond butter (2 Tbsp) and berries	23	1.7
Mexican Bowl with brown rice (1 cup), black beans (1 cup), salsa (¼ cup), avocado (1)	23	1.9
Amaranth breakfast bowl with amaranth (1 cup), soy milk (1 cup), walnuts (¼ cup), hemp seeds (2 Tbsp), berries	28	1.9
Teff wrap (1 wrap) with lentils (1 cup) and mixed veggies (carrots, spinach)	26	1.8
Oatmeal (1 cup), soy milk (1 cup), pecans (1.5 oz), hemp seeds (2 Tbsp), flax meal (2 Tbsp)	32	2.1
Tempeh Bolognese (4 oz tempeh, 1 cup lentil pasta, 1 cup red pasta sauce)	38	2.7

*Note: portion size can be increased if your needs are greater

Post-Exercise Recovery

In addition to fluid and electrolyte losses, training increases circulating hormones that break down glycogen and fat for fuel. These hormone levels remain high after exercise and continue to break down muscle tissue. Without adequate nutrient intake, this catabolic cascade continues for hours postexercise, contributing to muscle soreness and possibly compromising training adaptations and subsequent performance.

To repair and build muscle, athletes should refuel with high-protein foods (20–40 grams of protein) immediately following exercise, especially after resistance training. While it is crucial to replenish the body with protein and amino acids immediately after exercise, athletes should consume protein regularly throughout each day to stimulate whole-body protein synthesis for up to 48 hours after exercise.

Don't forget the carbohydrates! **Carbohydrates can prevent muscle from breaking down by stimulating the release of insulin.** Resistance training athletes have been shown to benefit from consuming carbohydrates and protein after strenuous workouts. One simple way to replenish immediately following a workout is through smoothies, which help to rehydrate athletes while providing both carbohydrates and protein for optimal recovery.

What About the Quality of Plant-Based Protein?

It is possible that vegans may need extra protein because proteins in some plant foods are not as well-absorbed as those from animal foods (10–15% less absorption). Therefore, some plant-based experts recommend that plant-based eaters consume 10–20 percent more plant-based protein than omnivores to ensure adequate protein intake. For example, a recreational female omnivore athlete may need approximately 51 grams of protein a day (0.8 per kg body weight) while a 140-pound vegan woman may need 55–61 grams of protein a day. That can be as simple as two tablespoons of hemp seeds or ¼ cup black beans.

Since plants are powered with so many phytonutrients that aid in performance, recovery, prevention of lifestyle diseases, consuming more plant-based protein means you get that much more healing nutrition.

As mentioned previously, there are twenty total amino acids, nine of which are essential for life. Plant foods that have been touted for being "complete" in all nine essential amino acids get their notoriety because they have sufficient amounts of all nine essential amino acids. Examples include whole soy foods, quinoa, peas, spirulina, chia seeds, amaranth, and buckwheat. More recently, pistachios made the list (go pistachios!).

Other plant-based foods still have all nine essential amino acids, but they may be a little low in one or two essential amino acids. For example, legumes (including lentils, beans, and peanuts), are an important part of a plant-based diet and contain plenty of lysine, an essential amino acid that has raised concern about falling short on a plant-based diet. However, they are lower in methionine and cysteine, two other additional amino acids. Other foods that are high in lysine include quinoa, amaranth, cashews, and pistachios. Grains on the other hand are low in lysine. If you were to only consume grains, you may be slighting yourself of lysine.

Lysine has been raised as a concern for those following a plant-based diet. **Can you get enough lysine on a plant-based diet?** Yes. A recent review analyzed several studies looking at the protein intake of vegans and found that lysine intake was higher (43 mg/kg) than what is recommended (30 mg/kg).

When you eat a variety of plant-based foods like lentils and grains you will receive all of the essential amino acids you need. Eating these foods within the same meal used to be recommended. This practice used to be called "complementing plant proteins" and would indicate that beans and rice, for example, be eaten together so that they form complete proteins by complementing each other. However, research shows that this is not necessary and that simply eating a variety of plants throughout the day is sufficient. This is because the body maintains a reserve pool of amino acids in the muscles, blood, and liver for later use. In other words, your body can do its own "complementing" with the amino acids that you eat throughout the day.

Protein intake of plant-based athletes is not necessarily a question of specific amino acid distributions but more likely one of the total caloric and protein intake.

Protein Before Bedtime

Pre-sleep whey protein intake has been shown to improve overnight muscle protein synthesis, muscle size and strength, and muscle recovery. Perhaps you are following a common recommendation of ingesting 30–40 grams of whey protein (dairy protein) immediately before bed to boost muscle synthesis and metabolic rate. While whey protein has been extensively studied in the past, pea protein has been more recently studied. One study examined the effects of whey and pea protein supplementation on physiological adaptations following 8-weeks of high-intensity functional training (HIFT) with four training sessions per week that included squats and deadlifts. Participants consumed 24 grams of either whey or pea protein before and after exercise on training days, and in-between meals on non-training days. The researchers concluded that ingestion of whey and pea protein produce similar outcomes in measurements of body composition, muscle thickness, force production, workout of the day performance and strength following 8 weeks of HIFT.

A randomized controlled study that included 161 males between the ages of 18 and 35 years, went through 12 weeks of resistance training on upper limb muscles. Subjects had to take 25 grams of whey protein, pea protein or placebo twice a day during the 12-week training period. The supplementation with pea protein promoted a greater increase of muscle thickness as compared to the placebo and especially for people starting or returning to a muscular strengthening. No difference was obtained between whey protein and pea protein. These studies are examples of how plant-based protein can produce the same results as animal-based protein.

In summary, from the International Society of Sports Nutrition:

- To build and maintain muscle mass, an overall daily protein intake in the range of 1.4–2 grams of protein per kg of body weight a day is sufficient for most exercising individuals.

- To maximize muscle synthesis in resistance training, it is generally recommended that 0.25 grams of high-quality protein per kg of body weight or 20–40 grams per serving be consumed.

- Strive for higher leucine content to maximize muscle growth (0.7—3 grams) in addition to a balance of other essential amino acids immediately following training.

- Distribute protein evenly, every 3–4 hours throughout the day.

- The optimal time period to ingest protein can be individualized, but the muscle building effects of exercise can generally last 24–48 hours.

- Attempting to meet protein needs through whole foods first by consuming a variety of protein-rich foods to ensure receiving all essential amino acids. Supplementation with protein powder can be a practical way of ensuring protein quality and quantity intake.

- Endurance athletes should focus on achieving adequate carbohydrate intake to promote optimal performance; the addition of protein may help to offset muscle damage and promote recovery.

- Pre-sleep protein intake (30–40 grams) may provide increases in overnight muscle protein synthesis.

More specific information on the protein content of certain plant foods can be found on page 218 in Tables and References.

CHAPTER 5

Fat

"The most tangible thing that I observed when I shifted my nutrition to 100% whole foods plant based was the reduced recovery time between workouts and long runs. As an ultramarathon runner, nutrition is a really crucial component to performance DURING your running, i.e. eating on the run. Becoming entirely plant-based had essentially ZERO effect on what I ate while racing and training because being plant based is NOT restrictive! The transition I made 13+ years ago to become plant based was astonishingly easy."

—Jackie Merritt, ultramarathoner, mom of two

Fat serves numerous functions in the body—from protecting organs to helping absorb nutrients to manufacturing hormones and providing a source of energy. These functions are very important for general health as well as for physical activity. While carbohydrates may be the focus for endurance athletes and protein for strength athletes, or maybe a little of both for a variety of reasons, fat deserves some love too. During lower to moderate intensity physical activities and physical activities performed for a long duration, fuel from fat can be the primary energy source. However, fat does not provide energy for quick bursts of speed.

Fat: The Basics

Fat, like protein and carbohydrates, is an important macronutrient that provides the body with energy, not to mention a key component in many other functions like protecting the skeletal and nervous systems. Fat also helps to make essential vitamins A, D, E, and K bioavailable. However, not all fats are equal and not all are beneficial. Some fats are better for health than others and may even promote good health. Dietary fat can be found in foods from both plants and animals.

Okay, hang tight, I am about to dive into my favorite class of all time, organic chemistry! (Just kidding. And if anyone ever tells you that is their favorite class of time, they are lying.) **In general, there are three types of fats: saturated, unsaturated, and trans fatty acids.** Unsaturated fats are further broken down into polyunsaturated fats and monounsaturated fats. All fats have a similar chemical structure, a chain of carbon atoms bonded to hydrogen atoms.

What makes one fat different from another is the length and shape of the carbon chain and the number of hydrogen atoms connected to the carbon atoms. Slight differences in structure create major differences in form and function. The word "saturated" refers to the number of hydrogen atoms attached to each carbon atom. The chain of carbon atoms holds as many hydrogen atoms as possible and is saturated with hydrogens. Unsaturated fats, sometimes called the healthier dietary fat, are in the form of monounsaturated or polyunsaturated. They differ from saturated fats by having fewer hydrogen atoms bonded to their carbon chains.

Trans fats occur when hydrogen is added to vegetable oil. **The process, called hydrogenation, causes the fat to solidify at room temperature.** Trans fats are also found naturally in some animal products like meat and dairy. Research shows that unsaturated fats may offer health benefits when replacing saturated or trans fats. *Phew*...okay, done with science class for the moment.

Fat Needs for Athletes

There are no specific dietary fat recommendations for athletes; therefore, the same recommendation given for the general adult population—consume 20–35% of total calories from fat—also applies to athletes. That said, individual requirements may vary between individuals. For example, elite endurance athletes may require a higher percentage of carbohydrates and less fat in their diet when compared to an athlete with a smaller training load. While individual needs may vary, the important point is that every athlete needs to include fat in their diet.

Fat plays many roles in an athlete's diet: from providing an energy source at lower training intensities to helping with absorption of essential vitamins to playing a part in synthesizing hormones.

Minimizing saturated and trans fats while focusing on monounsaturated and polyunsaturated fats is best as the latter types of fats have been shown to help with health and performance. What's more, saturated fat is more difficult to use as a fuel source, may disrupt the gut microbiome, and has been associated with cardiovascular disease.

A special nod to omega-3 fatty acids, types of polyunsaturated fats, which have been shown to have beneficial effects on athletes, including reducing muscle soreness and inflammation after training. Fat is slowly digested, which does not make for the ideal pre-training nutrient. That's why the time of day it is consumed during should be considered based on training and competition schedules. Consuming fat in meals separate from training is ideal. For example, including nuts in your morning oatmeal after you've trained or enjoying avocado on a sandwich at lunch, hours before your evening workout may be best for training.

Saturated Fat

Most saturated fat comes from animal sources like meat, poultry, and dairy. Palm oil, coconut oil, and cocoa butter are examples of plants that contain saturated fat. You can tell they are saturated because they are solid at room temperature. Eating too much saturated fat can increase total blood cholesterol levels and LDL cholesterol levels. A 2015 review of 15 randomized controlled trials looked at saturated fat and heart disease. The researchers concluded that replacing saturated fat in your diet with polyunsaturated fat from plants may reduce your heart disease risk.

While the impact of saturated fat on heart disease has been most often studied, there are other studies looking at saturated fat's effect on other health issues, like its ability to increase inflammation. **Inflammation is believed to play a central role in many of the chronic lifestyle diseases.** Over the years, research looking at the effect of saturated fat on inflammation in relation to our immune system has grown. Research shows that high-fat meals may promote endotoxins, which stimulate immune cells and lead to an inflammatory response. What affects this response is the amount and type of fat. There is evidence showing that saturated fat may induce an inflammatory response, while omega-3 fatty acids can reduce inflammation.

While research around fat's impact on gut health is still emerging, a recent systematic review found that saturated fat may negatively impact the gut microbiota and create an unhealthy metabolic state. Polyunsaturated fats, in the form of omega-3 fatty acids, have shown a positive impact on the gut by increasing gut bacteria diversity and reducing inflammation.

Saturated fat has also been associated with the incidence as well as the progression of prostate cancer and negative outcomes in women with breast cancer.

The Dietary Guidelines for Americans suggest that less than 10 percent of calories per day come from saturated fats. The American Heart Association recommends 5-6 percent of calories come from saturated fat.

Trans Fats

Trans fatty acids can appear naturally in the fatty portions of meat and dairy and also appear in foods that contain partially hydrogenated vegetable oils. Artificial trans-fat are in foods that contain partially hydrogenated oil. It's formed when hydrogen is added to liquid oil turning it into solid fat. Often, food manufacturers use artificial trans-fat in food products because it is inexpensive, and it increases the food's shelf life, stability, and texture. Foods that may contain artificial trans-fat include fried items, savory snacks (like microwave popcorn), frozen pizzas, baked goods, margarines and spreads, and coffee creamers. You might find trans-fat in fried foods like French fries and doughnuts, baked goods like cookies and cakes, and processed snack foods like crackers and popcorn. These types of fats are pretty terrible for your health and have been linked to high LDL cholesterol, heart disease, stroke and diabetes, as well as overall inflammation.

The Dietary Guidelines for Americans 2010 and the Institute of Medicine recommend that individuals should limit trans fatty acid consumption to less than 1 percent of calories. Even small amounts of trans fats can harm health: for every 2 percent of calories from trans-fat consumed daily, the risk of heart disease rises by 23 percent. That is a very little bit of trans fat in exchange for a huge impact on health.

Trans fat intake has significantly decreased in the U.S. as a result of efforts to increase awareness of its health effects through Nutrition Facts label changes, food manufacturers voluntarily reformulating foods, and restriction of its use in some restaurants and other food service outlets. Labeling laws allow food companies to round down to zero and claim "no trans fats" or "zero grams of trans fats" if the amount per serving is less than 0.5 g, despite still containing hydrogenated oils. Effective in 2020, the FDA banned the use of partially hydrogenated oils in processed foods, which should help to further decrease trans fat consumption.

Even with the efforts mentioned above, on average, Americans still consume 1.3 grams of artificial trans-fat each day. **To avoid trans fatty acids, the most important thing you can do is eat a diet rich in whole plant-based foods.** The second most important thing you can do is check the ingredient list on food labels to see if there is any partially hydrogenated oil in the product. If there is, put it back on the shelf.

Unsaturated Fats

Studies have consistently shown that eating foods with monounsaturated fat can improve cholesterol and decrease risk for cardiovascular disease. (Extra virgin cold-pressed olive oil and avocados are examples of monounsaturated fats that have been touted for their heart healthy benefits.) Eating foods rich in monounsaturated fat in place of saturated fat may improve blood cholesterol levels, which may decrease risk of heart disease and type 2 diabetes. Examples of whole foods high in monounsaturated fat include almonds, cashews, peanuts, pecans, olives, nut butters, and avocados.

The discovery that monounsaturated fat could be healthful came from the Seven Countries Study during the 1960's. It revealed that people in Greece and other parts of the Mediterranean region enjoyed a low rate of heart disease despite a high-fat diet. The main fat in their diet, though, was not the saturated animal fat common in countries with higher rates of heart disease. It was olive oil, which contains mainly monounsaturated fat. This finding produced a surge of interest in olive oil and the "Mediterranean diet," a style of eating regarded as a healthful choice today.

Although there is no recommended daily intake of monounsaturated fats, the Institute of Medicine recommends using them, along with polyunsaturated fats, to replace saturated and trans fats. Of note the Mediterranean diet is also packed with vibrant plant-based foods like fruits, vegetables, whole grains, and legumes, which also have a huge positive impact on health.

Polyunsaturated Fats

Polyunsaturated fats are known as "essential fats" because the body cannot make them and needs to get them from foods. Polyunsaturated fats are used to build cell membranes and the outer sheaths of nerves. They are needed for blood clotting, muscle movement, and to fight inflammation.

There are two main types of polyunsaturated fats: omega-3 fatty acids and omega-6 fatty acids. Both types offer health benefits, especially when replacing saturated fat. Eating polyunsaturated fats in place of saturated fats or highly refined carbohydrates may reduce LDL cholesterol, improve cholesterol profile, and lower triglycerides.

Plant-based foods and oils are the primary source of this fat. Polyunsaturated fat, in the form of omega-6 fatty acids, is found in tofu, nuts, seeds, vegetable oils, and margarines. Omega-3 fatty acids are types of polyunsaturated fat that have been shown to have health benefits on the heart, brain, blood pressure, and joints. Plant-based sources of omega-3 fatty acids include flax meal, chia seeds, hemp seeds, walnuts, and, while not as high as nuts and seeds, some leafy greens and Brussel sprouts also contain omega 3 fatty acids. The debatable issue with plant-based sources of omega-3's is the conversion rate to DHA and EPA.

The Importance of DHA and EPA

Omega-3 fatty acids play important roles in brain function, normal growth and development, and inflammation. Deficiencies have been linked to a variety of health problems, including cardiovascular disease, some cancers, mood disorders, arthritis, and more. However, that does not mean taking high doses translates to better health and disease prevention and not all omega-3 supplements are equal.

EPA (eicosapentaenoic acid) and DHA (docosahexaenoic acid) are types of omega-3 fatty acids that are abundant in fatty fish and algae. The body needs EPA & DHA omega-3 fatty acids to develop and function optimally from the time that we are born until the time we reach old age. During fetal development, EPA and DHA are important for proper formation of the nervous system, eyes, and immune system. (Moms may remember DHA and EPA in prenatal vitamins needed during pregnancy.) EPA and DHA may affect many aspects of cardiovascular function including inflammation and improving blood flow. These essential fatty acids have also been linked to promising results in cognitive function in those with very mild Alzheimer's disease and preventing mood disorders.

Fish and algae sources provide DHA and EPA directly, but what happens when you eat only plant-based foods and omit fish? **Vegetarians and vegans rely on the conversion of fats from walnuts, flax, and chia to these essential fatty acids.** Plant based foods contain what is called alpha-linolenic acid (ALA), an omega-3 fatty acid that is converted to EPA and DHA. Studies find that only 2–10 percent of ALA is converted to DHA and EPA. It is estimated that 5 percent to 10 percent of ALA is converted to EPA, but less than 2 percent to 5 percent of it is converted to DHA. This raises the question, do vegans and vegetarians get enough? There are many factors that can affect conversion rates like genetics, age, health status, poorly designed diets (can decrease conversion), ultra-high intake of omega-6 fatty acids (can reduce conversion by as much as 40–50 percent!), trans and saturated fat intake, fasting, protein deficiency, alcohol intake, and deficiencies of certain vitamins and minerals like B3, B6, magnesium, and zinc.

Interestingly, studies show that young women may convert ALA into DHA and EPA better than men. One study showed that young women converted up to 36 percent while in men, the conversion was a total of 16 percent. It may be that the higher conversion rate in young women is due to the need for extra EPA and DHA during child-bearing years. Bodies are so smart!

As mentioned above, the amount of omega-6 fatty acids can impact the conversion of ALA to DHA and EPA. The ratio of omega 6 fatty acids to omega 3 fatty acids may be a marker of health. Most western societies are sub optimally functioning with an omega 6 to omega 3 ratio of 15–16 to 1 when ideally, the ratio should be 4 to 1. To improve the omega 6 to omega 3 ratio, include omega 3-rich foods in your diet daily. Ground flax, chia seeds, hemp seeds, and walnuts are all rich sources of omega 3's. Add one or two tablespoons daily to smoothies, grain bowls, or oatmeal, and use flax meal or chia as your "egg" in baking (see recipes for ideas).

AMOUNT OF ALPHA-LINOLENIC ACID IN PLANT-BASED FOODS		
Food	Serving	Amount of alpha-linolenic acid (grams)
Brussel sprouts	1 cup	0.4
Chia seeds	2 tablespoons	4
Flax meal	2 tablespoons	3.2
Flaxseed oil	1 tablespoon	7.8
Flaxseed, whole	2 tablespoons	4.8
Greens, mixed	1 cup	0.1
Hemp seed, hulled	2 tablespoons	1.2
Hemp seed oil	1 tablespoon	2.8
Mustard oil	1 tablespoon	0.8
Tofu	½ cup	0.3
Walnuts	¼ cup	2.6

Adapted from Linus Pauling Institute and Today's Dietitian

Personally, I recommend an omega-3 fatty acid supplement to those following a whole food plant-based diet as reassurance. Receiving omega 3's from foods like chia and flax is important because of a whole foods first mindset, plus these foods offer so much nutrition in general. However, without knowing the exact conversation of their alpha linolenic acid to DHA and EPA, it is tough to say whether or not you are getting enough. There is a test called the Omega 3 Index that can show if your conversion from ALA to DHA and EPA is sufficient. If the test shows that your DHA and EPA levels are adequate, then you may not need supplementation. However, if the levels are low, or if you don't do the test, then I would recommend omega 3 supplementation.

Remember, this is supplemental. I like to think of it as a "top-off" to your diet. Adding just a little to ensure you are getting enough without being excessive. Look for algae-based sources of omega 3 fatty acids, third party testing (see chapter on supplements to learn more about what to look for in supplements), and 250–500 mg a day of DHA and EPA combined. You will typically find that DHA is in higher amounts. For example, Complement, a U.S.-based brand, has a plant-based omega 3 that contains 275 mg of DHA and 140 mg of EPA.

Here's the bottom line with fats:

- Strive for 20–35% of daily calories from fat.
- Limit saturated fat to less than 10 percent of total daily calories.
- Limit trans-fat to less than 1 percent of your daily calories.
- Incorporate food sources of omega 3's daily.

For athletes, reducing saturated and trans-fat, optimizing the omega 6 to omega 3 fatty acid ratio, and consuming whole food plant sources of fat may benefit athletes by reducing inflammation and helping to maintain proper vascular function, which may support athletic performance.

WHAT'S THE DEAL WITH OIL?

Most oils used in restaurants and food products have no nutritional benefits and may present health issues. For example, soybean and corn oils can be made from genetically engineered crops, they are highly processed as well as very high in omega-6 fatty acids.

The issue with olive oil and avocado oil is that they are processed and contain less nutrition than their whole food origins, olives, and avocado. For example, one whole avocado has almost 10 grams of fiber, lots of anti-inflammatory carotenoids, B vitamins, and vitamin E in addition to the fat and water content. When you remove only the fat to make avocado oil, you leave behind all of that nutrition that your body needs to function at its best. You are losing a lot of the brilliant nature. Nature combines these nutrients for a reason and our bodies were designed to work with these whole foods, not the broken-down pieces and extracts.

Same thing goes for olives and olive oil, corn and corn oil, or peanuts and peanut oil. In their whole food form, they offer so much nutrition, vitamins, minerals, phytonutrients, and fiber. The oil extracted from them may bring some beneficial compounds but significantly less than the whole food. Reducing oil consumption can help you achieve body composition goals if it is to lose body fat and it can also help to decrease inflammation. Not only will you improve your omega 6 to omega 3 ratio by limiting oil, but you are adding nutrient-dense foods in place of oil that work to reduce inflammation. For example, instead of using olive oil or avocado oil to make a dressing, use whole avocado in place of the oil. It adds lots of creaminess in addition to nutrition. Choosing to eat whole foods is a better option, getting your fats from nuts, avocados, and seeds over oil.

That said, if you are eating mostly whole food plant-based, a certain amount of these oils may be helpful in cooking. You just may want to ensure it's a high quality oil. I usually recommend cold-pressed extra virgin olive oil or flax oil, but flax seed oil should not be used for high heat cooking so either use it for low heat or a little drizzle over meals once the meal is cooked. For high heat cooking, avocado oil can be a good choice, but try to choose organic as many avocado oils may say it is avocado oil in the bottle but actually be a lesser quality oil or a blend of lesser quality oils.

CHAPTER 6

Fiber

"My diet is definitely more plant based now than it ever has been in my life. For me, a plant based diet has helped with feeling energized during my workouts, more focused during my training sessions, better at maintaining my goals during workouts—such as maximizing wattage output, hitting a time on a speed workout or reps during a lifting session. I also feel that it has helped with recovery time after strenuous exercise as far as gearing towards the food that I know will help reduce inflammation in the body."

—**Megan,** competitive runner and cyclist,
mom of four, neonatal nurse

Athletes may choose to consume low fiber foods to prevent gastrointestinal upset during training or competition. This results in low whole-food plant-based consumption, which is associated with reduced gut bacteria diversity and overall health in the general population. While there is little research on dietary fiber's effect on the microbiome in athletes, there is clear evidence in the general population that bacteria in the gut produce byproducts that can impact metabolism, immune function, inflammation, and mental health—all of which may be important for athletes. As more elite and everyday athletes suffer from psychological and gastrointestinal conditions that can be linked to the gut, plant-based diets are moving to the forefront.

The gastrointestinal tract contains more than 100 trillion microorganisms. Somewhere between 300 and 1000 different species live in the gut, with most estimates at about 500. Gut microbes digest fiber, producing energy, folate, vitamin K2, and short chain fatty acids, all essential for health. The gut microbiota also protects us from pathogens and carcinogens, influences intestinal motility, and supports the immune system. Research shows that the gut microbiota also influences neurotransmitters such as serotonin, GABA and dopamine, especially in response to physical and emotional stress.

Because the gut can play a large role in overall health and communicates with the nervous system (including the brain), it has been called the "second brain." **An imbalance of gut bacteria can disrupt the gut and, therefore, overall physical and mental health.** Lack of total fiber and lack of a variety of fiber can create an imbalance of gut bacteria.

One systematic review on endurance exercise and gut microbiota suggested that gut microbiota might have a key role in controlling the oxidative stress and inflammatory responses as well as improving metabolism, energy expenditure, and hydration during intense exercise. How does one build a healthy and diverse microbiota through diet? You may have guessed it: by eating a wide variety of plant-based foods that are packed with fiber and phytonutrients.

Fiber: The Basics

Dietary fiber is found in whole plant foods such as grains, vegetables, fruits, legumes, nuts, and seeds. In general, the least-processed choices are those that provide the most fiber.

By including whole, unprocessed plant-based foods at every meal, fiber recommendations can easily be met. Getting a healthy and diverse amount of fiber includes eating the following daily:

- A variety of vegetables from all of the vegetable subgroups including leafy greens, cruciferous vegetables, alliums and mushrooms and ensuring a rainbow of colors like greens, reds, oranges, purples and yellows.

- Legumes

- Whole grains

- Fruits

- Nuts and seeds

Tips for increasing fiber intake include:

- Replace refined processed foods with higher-fiber options (for example, substituting whole grain bread for white bread or brown rice for white rice).

- Include a serving of legumes each day (black bean burger, lentils on a salad, edamame snack).

- Layer meals with colorful fruits and vegetables (adding red onions on a sandwich, broccoli to a stir fry, or topping avocado toast with leafy greens and tomato).

- Ensure that there are at least three plant-based colors per meal.

Types of Fiber

When I went to school to become a dietitian, fiber was categorized into two categories: soluble and insoluble, with its main function being to move food through the digestive system. As science has progressed, we now know that fiber has many more roles than simply moving food through the gastrointestinal tract. This research has led to a change in fiber's identity, from simply soluble and insoluble to more specifically based on its physiological effects.

Soluble fiber includes viscous fiber that forms a gel in the intestinal tract, which has been shown to lower LDL (bad) cholesterol and slow absorption of carbohydrates into the bloodstream (reducing the rise in blood sugar after meals). Research also shows that soluble fiber can aid in weight management since it moves through our system slowly and can make us feel full quickly. Foods high in viscous fiber include oats, apples, beans, sweet potatoes, asparagus, Brussels sprouts, and barley.

Fermentable fibers, often referred to as prebiotics, are broken down by health-promoting gut bacteria to produce short-chain fatty acids called butyrate, acetate and propionate that have demonstrated a variety of health benefits such as transporting important minerals like iron, calcium, and magnesium. Through promotion of a healthy gut microbiome, research suggests that fermentable fiber could suppress development of chronic inflammation. Foods that are high in prebiotic fiber include dandelion, asparagus, bananas, apples, chicory root, Jerusalem artichokes, leeks, garlic, onion, jicama, millet, barley, oats, wheat bran, cocoa, flaxseeds, sweet potatoes, seaweed and more. There is not a specific recommendation for adequate intake of prebiotic fiber. Therefore, a diet that includes a diverse variety of fiber-rich fruits, vegetables, legumes, and whole grains has the most potential for obtaining adequate prebiotic fiber.

Insoluble fiber, also known as "bulking" fiber is the type of fiber that creates healthy stool. Another important function of bulking fiber is that it may provide long-term health protection by speeding passage of waste through the gut, diluting potential carcinogens, and reducing carcinogen exposure in the colon. This type of fiber can also help to prevent constipation. (There's nothing worse than being constipated during intense training or competition!) Foods high in insoluble fiber include leafy greens, nuts, seeds, beans, broccoli, carrots, and potatoes.

There is also isolated functional fiber like psyllium, beta-glucans, and wheat dextrin in supplements or an added ingredient in foods such as cereal, bread, snack bars, and yogurt. Some functional fibers occur naturally in plants (such as psyllium from the husk of psyllium seed or beta-glucan from oats or barley), while others are manufactured, including wheat dextrin formed by heat and acid treatment of wheat starch, and methylcellulose from chemically treated wood pulp. These are examples of soluble fiber that have been added to foods or sold individually as supplements and used to increase fiber for health benefits. There are also culinary uses for these fibers like replacing fat in food products, adding a crispy coating to foods, or replacing eggs in baking recipes that need a binder.

Fiber Needs for Athletes

At present, there are no specific dietary fiber recommendations for athletes due to the limited research being done in this area. **Therefore, athletes should follow the general population's recommendations.** Dietary reference intakes for dietary fiber are based on evidence that fiber reduces the risk of heart disease. The basic recommendation is 14 grams of fiber per 1,000 calories a day. Translated into Adequate Intake recommendations, women need a minimum of 25 grams of fiber a day and men need a minimum of 38 grams of fiber a day up to 50 years of age. For women and men over 50 years of age, the recommendations are 21 grams a day and 30 grams a day, respectively. Adequate Intakes for youth range from 19 to 38 grams per day based on age and gender.

As you start to increase your fiber intake, consider doing two things:

1. Increase fiber slowly.
2. Drink enough water.

With less than 5 percent of Americans getting adequate fiber in their diet, chances are that you may not be getting enough. Not to mention, bodybuilding athletes may limit carbohydrates and boost protein to optimize their physique, which can greatly disrupt the gut microbiome. Alternately, endurance athletes may opt for high glycemic, low fiber foods to fuel their training, which may result in low fiber intake.

What I'm trying to say is, assess your fiber intake and, if it's low, increase fiber slowly to prevent gastrointestinal discomfort. There is no hard rule for this, but I would suggest adding 5–10 grams per week to let your body adjust to the increase. You also might notice that you can tolerate certain high fiber foods better than others. **Before you try too hard to diversify your diet by adding several new foods that you have never before consumed, start slowly with the variety as well.** That way you can identify any particular food that does not agree with you. During this time, it may also be helpful to keep a food journal and document the foods you are consuming and how they affect you. Also, be patient. Sometimes it can take 2–6 weeks for your body to adjust to different types of fiber. You may experience some gassiness during this time, which could be a perfectly normal sign that the healthy bacteria are doing their job.

Another way to prevent abdominal gas, cramping and constipation is by drinking enough water as you increase your fiber intake. You want to do this as an athlete anyway, but a general rule of thumb is to drink enough water until your urine becomes clear. Another simple way to calculate basic water needs is to take your body weight and divide it by 2. For example, a 150-pound person will need 75 ounces (or about nine to ten 8-ounce cups) of water a day just for maintenance. If you exercise often, or sweat a lot, then you may need a higher intake. See the next chapter on hydration to get more details on how to adequately hydrate.

A DEEPER LOOK AT PREBIOTICS AND PROBIOTICS

Prebiotic fiber is a non-digestible carbohydrate (or simply a type of fiber) that fuel healthy gut bacteria and help support a healthy microbiome balance. Basically, prebiotics are food for beneficial bacteria that live in us. Since your body cannot completely break down prebiotics, they pass through your digestive system to the colon where they are fermented by your gut microflora. This fermentation process feeds the friendly bacteria in your gut, helping them to produce essential nutrients, including short-chain fatty acids such as butyrate, acetate, and propionate, which nourish the digestive system. The fermentation process also helps improve mineral absorption, production of vitamin K and boost overall health.

By feeding healthy bacteria in our gut, prebiotics may support digestion, improve immunity, decrease inflammation, support bone health, assist with metabolism, balance hormones, relieve stress and anxiety, and boost mood.

On the other side, the International Scientific Association for Probiotics and Prebiotics defines **probiotics** as live microorganisms that, when administered in adequate amounts, confer a health benefit on the host. Probiotics are naturally found in our intestines. It is estimated that over 500 different bacterial strains live in the human gut. A lack of diversity in probiotic strains has been linked to obesity, digestive issues, and many other health issues.

Probiotics can colonize the gut and produce health benefits like neutralizing toxins, producing short chain fatty acids, boosting mineral absorption, synthesizing vitamins, and making the gut barrier stronger.

Fermented foods such as miso, sauerkraut, kimchi, plant-based yogurt and kefir, may contain probiotics. To ensure store bought products contain beneficial probiotics, look for "live cultures" on the food label, as not all fermented foods contain probiotics.

Prebiotics and probiotics work synergistically. While prebiotics are non-digestible foods for our gut, probiotics are live microorganisms that feed on prebiotics. Prebiotics and probiotics work together, keeping the gut healthy and communicating with other systems keeping our whole body healthy and mind clear.

Now, to put this into practice. **Synbiotics** are prebiotic and probiotic compounds mixed together, either in food or supplemental form. It makes sense, since they work together, that they would be together for optimal health. For healthy individuals, I personally recommend optimizing gut health naturally through whole plant-based foods.

That means following the following recommendations:

- Eat at least 30–40 grams of fiber a day from a variety of plant-based foods (fruits, vegetables, legumes, whole grains, nuts, and seeds).

- Incorporate a variety of prebiotic foods daily as a part of total fiber intake (cook with garlic, add onion to a sandwich, include asparagus in your stir fry or eat oatmeal in the morning).

- Add 1–2 tablespoons of a probiotic food to your diet daily (add kimchi to avocado toast, add sauerkraut to a sandwich, make a miso sauce or salad dressing to use throughout the week or snack on probiotic-rich coconut yogurt daily).

- Drink plenty of water.

The Role of the Microbiome in Athletes

It is known that exercise can have anti-inflammatory effects throughout the body, prevent chronic lifestyle diseases, and contribute to more efficient carbohydrates metabolism. It is also known that being sedentary can lead to lifestyle diseases such as obesity, heart disease, and diabetes. Recent evidence supports the microbiome's role in prevention of these diseases and emerging research is supporting the role of exercise diversifying the microbiota. **Exercise can influence the gut microbiome, which can affect athletic performance as well as immune function, lowering susceptibility to infection,** inflammatory response, and tissue repair. Maintaining a healthy gut microbiota is essential for an athlete's overall health, training, and performance. It has been noted across several studies that athletes have increased gut microbial diversity compared with more sedentary individuals.

One study looked at 40 male rugby players compared to 46 sedentary people. They found that the rugby players had enhanced amino acid and carbohydrates metabolism. They also produced more short chain fatty acids. It was a small study, but the researchers speculated that the athletes had better fitness and overall health than the control group due to a more diverse microbiota.

A subsequent study of the same population concluded that athletes had a higher abundance of short-chain fatty acids (SCFA), the substances produced by bacteria in the gut that play a part in overall health.

It was also observed that routine exercise is proportional to the amount of Prevotella, a bacteria associated with increased branched-chain amino acid (BCAA) pathways, which is important in muscle recovery. An increase in another bacteria, *Methanobrevibacter smithii*, has been linked to more adenosine triphosphate (ATP), or energy, creation in amateur cyclists.

Another study discovered that one type of bacteria called Veillonella was enriched in the gut microbiome of marathon runners, compared to non-runners. This type of bacteria has been associated with improved performance.

With regard to diet, one study compared the gut microbiome of bodybuilders, distance runners and control subjects. Each of the groups ingested a different sport specific diet. Results suggest that high-protein diets may have a negative impact on gut microbiota diversity for athletes. It also showed that resistance training athletes who follow a high protein, low carbohydrates diet had decreased short chain fatty acids.

Exercise clearly plays a part in diversifying the microbiota. **Eating a plant-based diet with a variety of fiber, including prebiotics, and fermented foods with probiotics may optimize gut health, which may reduce inflammation and impact overall athletic performance.** What you eat determines which bacteria are able to thrive in your gut. Research tells us that good bacteria could get stronger when fed colorful, fibrous plant-based foods.

CHAPTER 7

Hydration

"I do an active workout 4–5 times per week. This past weekend, I did a strenuous short hike with a steep elevation. Before I went vegan and plant based, I would always be sore the same evening I did the hike and into the next morning. Since going fully plant-based, I find that my recovery is quick. I don't have the same soreness and can jump into a new workout easier the next day. Also, I am sleeping much better since my body is less sore, which used to wake me up at night."

—**Alan,** hiker, runner, Los Angeles, CA

I can speak firsthand to hydration dilemmas. When I was in my twenties, I trained pretty hard between cycling and running. Being young, naive and a bit careless at times, I did not always properly hydrate. I would wake up early before work to go for a 4–6 mile run and could immediately tell the days when I was properly hydrated and days when I neglected to drink enough water the previous day and did not have at least two glasses of water before running out the door. My performance suffered greatly. I would feel like I was treading muddy water. My joints felt like they were about to crack and my neck and back would ache during the run. I would also be a cranky monster.

Hydration not only affects performance, but it affects rate of injury, ability to focus, mood and recovery. I still run once or twice a week with yoga practice being my daily form of exercise. I have noticed that dehydration affects my yoga practice as well. (I know, right? You might think I would be wiser with age, but dehydration is sneaky like that and can easily creep up on you!) Days that I am dehydrated lead to muscle soreness and tightness, as well as body aches and pains. Hydration helps joints, ligaments, and tendons to be lubricated and move more freely, whether it is yoga, running, cycling, or gardening. There is evidence to suggest that hydration might be one of the most important predictors of exercise performance.

Hydration and Athletic Performance

Hydration is one of the most important nutritional concerns for an athlete. Why is fluid so important during exercise? Approximately 60–70 percent of body weight is water. **Water has many important roles in the body, which includes maintaining blood volume and regulating body temperature.** During exercise, the body cools itself by sweating, which results in a loss of body fluid. Fluid is also lost through the lungs while breathing. If the fluid is not replaced, dehydration can follow. Sweat production (fluid loss) increases with increasing ambient temperature and humidity, as well as with an increase in exercise intensity. It is important to replace fluid at regular intervals during practice or competition otherwise to prevent dehydration from creeping up on you.

Dehydration can result in decreased blood volume which can lead to:

- Decreased amount of blood pumped with each heartbeat
- Lack of oxygen to the muscles
- Decreased performance
- Decreased elimination of metabolic by-products (causing toxin build-up)
- Exhaustion
- Crankiness (unofficially added by my own personal experience!)

Both physical and mental performance decline as dehydration increases. Heart rate and body temperature increase, as well as the perception of how hard the exercise feels, especially when exercising in the heat. Skill level can be impaired, along with mental fatigue that can impact concentration and decision making—all important aspects of training and competition. Dehydration can also cause nausea, vomiting, diarrhea, and other gastro-intestinal problems during and after exercise. As you can see, it is important to hydrate!

Optimal hydration is dependent on a variety of factors but can generally be defined during exercise as avoiding fluid losses greater than 2–3 percent of body mass while also avoiding overhydration. Research has shown that losing as little as 2 percent of total body weight in sweat can negatively affect athletic performance. To give you an example, 2 percent of a 150-pound athlete is three pounds. If a 150-pound athlete loses three pounds during competition or training, their ability to perform at peak performance is impacted. Proper fluid replenishment during training and competition is key in preventing dehydration, optimizing performance, and reducing the risk of heat injury in athletes.

HYDRATION AND SWEATING

If you tend to sweat quite a bit during training, it might be helpful to note your sweat rate. Sweat rates vary between individuals, therefore, knowing your unique sweat rate and how much fluid you should be drinking is important as fluid needs are individual and rely on factors such as personal sweat rate, exercise mode, exercise intensity, environmental conditions, and exercise duration. Several factors contribute to sweat rate including temperature, humidity, clothing, and air flow. For example, individuals exercising in hot-humid environments with direct sunlight and minimal airflow will produce quite a bit of sweat and be at the greater risk of dehydration compared to individuals exercising in cooler temperatures with shade.

Also, the type of sport may influence individual needs. For example, sports that require uniforms and heavy equipment may impair the ability to optimize hydration during activity. Clothing provides insulation and presents a barrier to heat loss, resulting in increased sweat rates. For example, football players are at greater risk of body fluid loss compared to similar activities in which clothing is minimal. Athletes playing in hot and humid temperatures combined with heavy clothing and equipment need to pay special attention to hydration needs.

There are several ways to measure sweat rate. Here is a simple calculation from TruSport.org:

First, compare the difference in your weight (in pounds) before and after exercise. Multiply this by 16 to convert this figure to ounces. Now, record the amount of fluids (in ounces) consumed during the exercise and add it to your original figure. Divide this new total by the duration of your exercise (in hours) to find your sweat rate per hour.

Here's an example of what this looks like:

Weight before exercise (140 pounds) – weight after exercise (138 pounds) = 2 pounds
Weight loss (in pounds) x 16 ounces = 32 ounces
Amount of fluids consumed during activity = 16 ounces
Total fluids used during activity (32 + 16) = 48 ounces
Duration of activity, in hours = 2 hours
Sweat rate = 48 / 2 = 24 ounces per hour

Sports with specific rules, such as "stop-start" sports create their own unique hydration challenges. For example, soccer includes two 45-minute halves in which the ability to hydrate is extremely limited to players. At the other extreme are sports like baseball, basketball and tennis that include frequent rest breaks within playing time (e.g., time outs, change of ends or player rotations), allowing for fluids to be consumed through-out play time. **As you can see, an athlete's drinking strategy for a competition is unique to their sport.** To stay hydrated, it is important to plan ahead and ensure that there is plenty of water or other palatable fluids readily accessible. Also, monitor daily changes in weight, urine color and thirst to determine hydration during training and competition.

Preventing Dehydration

The number one way to prevent dehydration is to maintain body fluid levels by consuming plenty of fluids before, during, and after a workout or competition. Often, athletes do not realize that they are impacting performance as they become dehydrated. One group of scientists, Cheuvront and Kenefick, established three criteria to monitor early morning hydration:

- Body weight changes greater than 1 percent
- A conscious desire for water (thirst)
- Dark-colored urine

Two of these factors combined suggest daily fluid intake is likely inadequate, while all three factors indicate that daily fluid intake is very likely inadequate. You will want to know your baseline body weight to determine the percentage of weight change.

Urine color. The color of your urine first thing in the morning is an overall indicator of hydration status. Straw colored urine is a sign of appropriate hydration. Darker colored urine indicates dehydration. Bright urine often is produced soon after consuming vitamin supplements.

Sweat loss. Change in body weight before and after exercise is used to estimate sweat loss. Since an athlete's sweat loss during exercise is an indicator of hydration status, athletes are advised to follow customized fluid replacement plans that consider thirst, urine color, fluid intake, sweat loss and body weight changes that occur during exercise.

Waiting for thirst as an indication of hydration is not a good idea as by the time you feel thirsty, you are already deep into hydration and will have to play catch up hydrating. Interesting fact—many individuals do not feel thirsty until more than 2 percent of their body weight is lost. Waiting until you are thirsty can greatly impact your performance.

Below are guidelines for fluid replacement from the National Athletic Trainers Association, the Academy of Nutrition and Dietetics, and the American College of Sports Medicine.

- **Before Exercise:** Start exercise well hydrated. Athletes should drink 16–24 ounces of water within the 2 hours prior to training. At 10–20 minutes prior to exercise consume another 7–10 fl. oz. of water.

- **During Exercise:** Athletes should consume approximately 6–12 ounces every 10–20 minutes throughout their training. Drink beyond your thirst!

- **After Exercise:** It is recommended for athletes to record their weight before and after training. This is especially true in hot & humid conditions, in extreme cold weather training, for individuals with a high sweat rate, as well as high altitude. Athletes should replace every 1 pound loss in weight with 16–24 fluid ounces of water. The total fluid consumed should be focused within 2 hours post-training, however fully consumed within 6 hours.

Finally, know the signs of dehydration:

1. Thirst
2. Constipation
3. Unclear thinking
4. Mood changes
5. Flushed skin
6. Fatigue
7. Decreased exercise capacity
8. Increased body temperature during exercise
9. Faster breathing and pulse rate during exercise
10. Increased perception of effort during exercise

Fluid Replacement Drinks

Water is the best replacement fluid for exercise and sports that are low intensity and for shorter periods of time. Sports drinks may be useful during high intensity or endurance sports. Sports drinks containing between 6–8 percent of carbohydrates can provide energy to the working muscle that water cannot, which may increase exercise capacity and improve performance. A 6 percent solution contains about 14 grams of carbs per 8 fluid ounces. Studies show that carbohydrates ingestion through a sports drink can improve sport performance, especially when training lasts longer than 60–90 minutes of continuous activity. Athletes who consume a sports drink can maintain blood glucose levels at a time when muscle glycogen stores are diminished. This allows carbohydrates use for energy production to continue at high rates. Research has also shown that mouth rinses with carbohydrates can improve performance at rates similar to ingestion. Beverages containing more than one kind of sugar (i.e., glucose and fructose) can optimize carbohydrates absorption rates because each sugar is absorbed via different channels.

Replacing electrolytes is important when training or competing for more than two hours. Sodium is the predominant electrolyte lost via our sweat. One of its most important functions is to assist our cells in retaining the fluids we consume. Athletes who train or compete for more than two hours or who have high sweat losses, should replace both fluid and sodium during exercise. The ingestion of sodium during exercise may help with maintenance or restoration of blood plasma volume during exercise and recovery.

Recent research has suggested that a 6–8 percent carbohydrates sport drink with at least 110 mg of sodium per 8 ounce serving empties from the stomach just as fast as plain water. Endurance activities lasting longer than three hours may require as much as 175 mg of sodium per 8 ounce serving. There has been concern by some that sports drinks may contain too much sodium. However, many fluid replacement drinks are actually pretty low in sodium. An 8-ounce serving of a fluid replacement drink can have a sodium content similar to that of a cup of plant-based milk.

What NOT to Drink

It is not recommended to consume beverages with a carbohydrates content higher than 8 percent, which will slow the rate of fluid absorption in your body. During training, if the fluid you consume does not reach your body's cells, dehydration can occur. Some items which have more than 8 percent carbohydrates content include fruit juices, sodas, and carbohydrates gel. Beverages containing caffeine and carbonation are discouraged during training because they can stimulate excess urine production which can lead to dehydration.

However, studies do show that 1–2 six-ounce cups of coffee in the two hours before training may positively affect performance due to the caffeine. That said, caffeine in excess is on the NCAA Banned Substance List. For example, a urinary caffeine exceeding 15 micrograms per milliliter (about 500 milligrams or the equivalent of six to eight cups of brewed coffee, two to three hours before competition) can result in a positive drug test.

Of note, energy drinks may contain unlabeled or unclear amounts of banned stimulants like synephrine, which, when added to unknown amounts of caffeine, can result in serious health consequences, and can even be fatal. Read the ingredient label before scooping up something that claims instant energy.

Overhydration

Just like anything, over-consumption is not always a good thing. In cool weather or when the exercise intensity is low, sweat losses may be small. Drinking more fluid than necessary can interfere with performance and potentially be dangerous to health in several ways. Over-hydration during exercise can result in hyponatremia (low sodium levels), which is when the sodium levels get diluted in the bloodstream from excessive water consumption. Symptoms of hyponatremia include headaches, disorientation and in severe cases, coma, or death. It is important to note, however, that overhydration to this extreme is rare and dehydration is the more common issue for athletes.

However, if you are a slower athlete choosing to compete in endurance events over prolonged distances or duration, you may have the ability to drink much more than your true fluid needs, making you at potential risk of developing hyponatremia. If you happen to fall into this category, know that over hydrating is a thing and plan ahead to determine your fluid needs before event day.

KEY MICRONUTRIENTS

CHAPTER 8

Calcium

There are three common questions that come to people's mind when thinking about eating more plant-based foods or going completely plant-based:

- How do I get enough protein?
- Will I be deficient in iron if I don't eat meat?
- How do I get calcium if I cut out dairy?

These are valid questions. After all, we have been taught that protein comes from animal products, meat is a good source of iron, and milk is needed for strong bones. The meat and dairy industries have done a fantastic job over the years marketing these concepts to us, our parents, and the healthcare industry. However, there are many other foods that contain all of these nutrients.

By now you are well-versed in the protein arena and aware of the various ways you can get protein on a plant-based diet, but what about calcium? Before we dive into plant-rich sources of calcium, let's first talk about calcium's function, because it goes beyond bones.

Calcium: The Basics

Calcium is a mineral found in a variety of foods. It is important for bones as 99 percent of the calcium in the body is stored in bones and teeth, which helps to keep them strong by supporting their structure and durability. Calcium is also important for transmitting nerve impulses, clotting blood, contracting muscles, regulating blood pressure, and assisting with heart function.

Every day, we lose calcium through our skin, nails, hair, sweat, and urine. Athletes who are heavy sweaters lose even more calcium. **Our body cannot produce its own calcium, which is why it is important to get enough calcium from the food we eat.** When we do not get the calcium from food, it is taken from our bones which can cause bone weakening, loss and eventually may lead to fractures and broken bones.

Calcium and Athletic Performance

Because of calcium's role in bone health, muscle contraction, nerve transmission, and heart health, calcium is clearly important for vegan athletes. Not to mention, athletes who sweat a lot during training and competition may lose more calcium through perspiration. However, research on calcium needs in athletes is limited. It is suggested that athletes should strive for the RDA, but, of course, each individual athlete is different depending on age, gender, sport, and other lifestyle factors.

Calcium Needs for Athletes

The National Academy of Medicine, which establishes the RDA and the World Health Organization both recommend 1,000 mg of calcium per day for adults 19 to 50 years of age and 1200 mg for those over 50 years of age. However, it is not only the amount that matters most. What also matters is how much calcium is absorbed.

The absorption of calcium from food varies quite a bit. For example, the calcium absorbed from dairy milk is about 30 percent. The calcium absorption from soy milk is comparable to that of dairy milk, about 30 percent. However, other plant-based foods can range from 5 percent absorption to 65 percent absorption. For example, spinach, which is a good source of calcium, contains a compound called oxalates, which are crystals that plants create to protect themselves against predators and environmental elements. Oxalates bind minerals, like calcium, making them less available to us when we eat foods high in oxalates. Therefore, the absorption of calcium in spinach is only about 5 percent or less.

Cooking can reduce some of the oxalates but not very much. On the other hand, kale, which is an excellent source of calcium, is very low in oxalates. The absorption of calcium from kale is 60–65 percent. Spinach and kale are both great, nutrient-dense foods, but if you are trying to maximize calcium intake through daily leafy greens then opt for kale on most days. Other high oxalate leafy greens include beet greens, dandelion, and chard. Kale, mustard greens, collards, and broccoli are good sources of calcium and low in oxalates, so we absorb calcium from these foods very well.

Here's a tip: If you are drinking plant-based milk and want to maximize calcium intake then make sure to shake the carton well as the vitamins and minerals can settle to the bottom. Also, look for calcium fortified plant milk.

Beans can be a good source of calcium, however, there is the absorption factor again. Beans, like spinach, contain compounds that inhibit calcium absorption (as well as other minerals like zinc and iron) called phytates and lectins. Soaking, sprouting and fermenting beans can significantly reduce the phytate and lectin level, making calcium and other minerals more available. The same goes for nuts. Soaking them may lower these compounds and increase the bioavailability of minerals.

Other plant-based foods that are good sources of calcium include almonds, Brazil nuts, chia seeds, flax meal, sesame seeds, seaweed, amaranth, bok choy, Brussel sprouts, oranges, and fortified orange juice.

For more information on the calcium content of specific foods, please see page 220 under Tables and References at the end of this book.

Calcium Supplementation

If you do not eat calcium-rich foods often or are worried about meeting calcium needs, you might consider taking a calcium supplement. Note that it is a "supplement" meant to complement your diet, not provide 100 percent of your calcium needs. **It is still important to aim for optimal calcium intake from whole foods since whole foods provide other essential nutrients and also because calcium supplementation is not without side effects.** Supplementation may cause constipation, gas and bloating if taken in excess. Minimize side effects and maximize absorption by taking calcium with food and in smaller doses throughout the day. For example, split a 500 mg supplement into two 250 mg doses with meals twice a day.

THE RISK OF CALCIUM SUPPLEMENTS

While many studies show the benefit of calcium supplementation for bone health, there may be a link between high-dose calcium supplements and heart disease in women. A meta-analysis, released in 2010 and reviewing 11 studies, showed that women taking more than 500 mg a day of supplemental calcium, without vitamin D supplementation, had an increased incidence of heart attacks than did those taking the placebo. While it is not definitive, it shows that getting sufficient calcium from food should be the first line of defense to support bone health. Calcium supplementation may be warranted in those not receiving enough from food, but doses should be individualized, and excess doses should be avoided.

A similar controversy surrounds calcium and prostate cancer. Some studies have shown that high calcium intake from dairy products and supplements may increase risk, whereas another more recent study showed no increased risk of prostate cancer associated with total calcium, dietary calcium, or supplemental calcium intakes.

For both associations, the evidence is mixed, and more research is needed. Until more is known about these possible risks, it is important to be careful to avoid excessive amounts of calcium. As with any health issue, it is important to talk to your healthcare provider to determine what's right for you.

Calcium: The Bottom Line

To meet calcium requirements, vegan athletes should consume a variety of plant-based sources of calcium such as beans, leafy greens, tofu, nuts and seeds in sufficient quantities and consume more low-oxalate leafy greens. Choosing calcium-fortified foods such as calcium-fortified plant-based milks and fruit juices is also a suitable way to meet calcium needs. If you are not meeting calcium requirements through whole and fortified foods, then consider taking a calcium supplement to meet your calcium needs. Splitting the supplement 250–300 mg per dose, consumed with meals is recommended. Remember, food first and take a supplement only to meet your needs, if warranted.

CHAPTER 9

Vitamin D

Vitamin D deficiency is common, and not just among plant-based eaters. About one *billion* people worldwide have vitamin D deficiency and 50 percent of the population has vitamin D insufficiency. Vitamin D deficiency is associated with osteoporosis, increased risk of falls and fractures. Vitamin D insufficiency is defined as serum levels of 20–30 ng/mL and vitamin D deficiency as serum levels below 20 ng/mL. Although more research is needed, recent studies are showing an association between vitamin D deficiency and cancer, cardiovascular disease, diabetes, immune function, autoimmune diseases, and depression. Sixty percent of the elderly population in the United States are deficient in vitamin D.

Other than the aging population, people at most risk for vitamin D deficiency include those with:

- Higher skin melanin content
- Limited sun exposure (due to altitude, skin coverage or being indoors during sun hours)
- Malabsorption syndromes of the gastrointestinal tract
- Chronic liver disease
- Insufficient dietary intake
- Obesity

Vitamin D: The Basics

Vitamin D, also referred to as calciferol, is a fat-soluble vitamin that is naturally present in just a handful of foods, added to other foods, and available as a dietary supplement. It is also produced in our body when our skin is exposed to ultraviolet (UV) rays from the sunlight. Because our body can produce vitamin D when exposed to sunlight, it is also referred to as a hormone (hormones are synthesized in our bodies).

Since it is a fat-soluble vitamin, it should be accompanied by a fat source when taken orally for the best absorption. While water-soluble vitamins are excreted and not stored in the body, vitamin D and other fat-soluble vitamins (vitamins A, E, and K) accumulate in fatty tissues throughout your body and can be toxic if taken in large doses. Vitamin D does help your body absorb calcium, however too much vitamin D can create excess calcium to accumulate in the blood causing hypercalcemia which leads to digestive distress, fatigue, and bone loss.

The good thing is that this can only happen with excess vitamin D supplements. An overdose of vitamin D from too much sun is not possible as the body is pretty remarkable at regulating the amount you need converted from sun exposure.

The Role of Vitamin D

Vitamin D promotes calcium absorption in the gut and helps the body to maintain adequate serum calcium and phosphate concentrations. Vitamin D and vitamin K also work together to regulate calcium metabolism, which is essential for heart health. As you may know, vitamin D also plays a key role in bone health and strength. Without sufficient vitamin D, bones can become thin and brittle. Vitamin D sufficiency prevents rickets in children and osteomalacia (softening of the bones) in adults. Together with calcium, vitamin D helps protect older adults from osteoporosis. Vitamin D also controls the reduction of inflammation and plays a part in cell growth, neuromuscular and immune function, and glucose metabolism. As you can see, its role goes well beyond bones!

Vitamin D for Athletes

There is a high prevalence of vitamin D deficiency in athletes, which may increase risk of stress fractures, illness, and delayed muscle recovery. Deficiencies or insufficiencies have been found in dancers, taekwondo fighters, jockeys, elite wheelchair athletes, handball players, track and field athletes, weightlifters, swimmers, and volleyball players. Athletes training indoors may be especially susceptible to inadequate vitamin D, however research shows that it is not just indoor athletes that demonstrate low levels of vitamin D. Athletes with subtherapeutic vitamin D levels may be at higher risk of missing practices and games as a result of stress fractures, muscle injuries, and upper respiratory tract infections.

Recent research on athletes shows that vitamin D plays a role in muscle contraction and synthesis as well as athletic performance. The active form of vitamin D stimulates protein synthesis and the number of type II muscle cells, both of which lead to increased muscle contraction and strength. Researchers are finding that vitamin D deficiency may have a negative impact on muscle strength, power, and work, as well as overall performance.

Vitamin D insufficiency in athletes is associated with a higher frequency of diseases, including common colds, the flu, and gastrointestinal infections. In athletes, the incidence of respiratory diseases is higher, especially in elite athletes. Low levels of vitamin D may make professional athletes more susceptible to upper respiratory tract infections as individuals with higher levels of vitamin D show a lower propensity to them. Studies have shown that the incidence of upper respiratory tract infections increases in athletes with low vitamin D levels, especially during high-intensity exercise or prolonged and strenuous training periods.

Increasing Vitamin D Intake

If you are able, it's best to let the beautiful sun do its job by naturally providing vitamin D—not too much and not too little. However, if sun is not an option (or if you know your vitamin D levels are low), here are the currently supported recommendations:

RECOMMENDED DAILY AMOUNT OF VITAMIN D		
Age	Male	Female
14–18 years	15 mcg (600 IU)	15 mcg (600 IU)
19–50 years	15 mcg (600 IU)	15 mcg (600 IU)
51–70 years	15 mcg (600 IU)	15 mcg (600 IU)
>70 years	20 mcg (800 IU)	20 mcg (800 IU)

Adequate Intake (AI) from https://ods.od.nih.gov/factsheets/VitaminD-HealthProfessional/

In foods and dietary supplements, vitamin D has two main forms: D2 (ergocalciferol) and D3 (cholecalciferol). They differ slightly in their structures, but both forms are absorbed well in the small intestine. That said, vitamin D3 has been shown to increase and maintain serum levels of vitamin D in the blood more so than D2. Vitamin D is in its inactive state when it is absorbed in the intestines then converted to its active form in the liver and kidneys. (One reason why people with liver and kidney disease may have low vitamin D is because of their inability to convert the inactive to the active form.)

There are three ways to get vitamin D: sunshine, food, and supplementation.

Sunshine

In the case of vitamin D, sunshine is your best friend. The sun is the best way to naturally get vitamin D and it is important to get that exposure on bare skin without sunscreen. Wait, haven't we been told to avoid the sun if we want to minimize the risk of skin cancer and preserve aging skin?

The good news is that you do not have to spend hours in the sun for your body to achieve optimal vitamin D levels. Recommendations for time in the sun do vary depending on individual factors like skin pigmentation, age, the latitude of where you live (there is less direct sunlight further from the equator), skin cancer risk, and the season. Recommendations typically range from 10–30 minutes per day, without sunscreen, over a large portion of your body. Studies have found that people with dark skin pigmentation may need up to six times more sun exposure than people with light skin to get the same vitamin D3 production from their skin.

Food

The second optimal choice to obtain vitamin D is through food. However, natural vitamin D is found in only a handful of foods, most of which are animal-derived like certain types of fatty fish (halibut, salmon, and mackerel), animal organ meats like liver, and just a tiny amount in eggs and dairy products. Because they come with health risk factors and they are not environmentally friendly, I do not recommend animal-based products with vitamin D. Vitamin D can also be found in fortified foods like fortified orange juice, cereals, plant-based milk and light-exposed mushrooms.

PLANT-BASED MILK

A common question is which plant-based milk is best since there are so many options from cashew to almond to soy to hemp to oat. Other than opting for the flavor and texture that you love most, I suggest looking at the Nutrition Facts label to see which milk is fortified with important nutrients like calcium and vitamin D. Using plant-based milk is a great opportunity to boost intake of these nutrients. The amount of vitamins and minerals the milk contains can often be the differentiating factor when it comes to comparing nutrition between milk varieties.

The only plant-based foods that naturally contain vitamin D are certain types of mushrooms, as vitamin D2. Mushrooms can manufacture vitamin D in the same way as humans, exposure to sunlight (mushrooms are cool like that!). The vitamin D content of mushrooms can be increased either by exposing them to direct sunlight or using UV lamps during their growing process. If the mushrooms naturally contain vitamin D, it may say it on the packaging. Now, I know there are some hard-core naturalists out there. I totally understand, if there is a way to get nutrients from food in a sustainable, cruelty-free way, then I am all for it. However, I would not recommend relying on mushrooms as your sole source of vitamin D on a plant-based diet.

Supplements

If you know your vitamin D is low and you want to raise your vitamin D levels, the most reliable way to do so is to take a supplement. As mentioned above, there are two main forms of vitamin D: vitamin D2 and vitamin D3. While they are both effectively absorbed into the bloodstream from your intestines, your liver metabolizes vitamin D3 more effectively than D2, giving vitamin D3 the advantage as an effective supplement. Many of the vitamin D supplements come in gel, oil, or capsule form accompanied with a fat source. Depending on your vitamin D levels, anywhere between 600 IUs to 2000 IUs a day may be recommended. If your serum vitamin D level is extremely low, then you may be prescribed a higher dose until your serum levels normalize at which time you may only need a maintenance dose.

Most vitamin D supplements come in the form of vitamin D3, or cholecalciferol. Traditionally, vitamin D3 was sourced from sheep lanolin, making it obviously non-vegan or plant-based. **However, more recently, due to consumer demand, vegan vitamin D3 supplements are readily available.** The plant-based version of D3 is sourced from lichen, an organism that comes from algae or cyanobacteria. You may see vitamin D as part of a multivitamin or paired with a handful of other vitamins and minerals like vitamin K and calcium since they work together.

If you are taking supplements to raise low serum vitamin D levels, follow up with your healthcare provider to determine the best time to get tested again. If your levels normalize, you may need a lower maintenance supplemental dose, but that can only be determined by knowing your numbers.

Vitamin D: The Bottom Line

Future research on vitamin D's role in athletes is still being carried out. For now, it is recommended that vitamin D levels are checked at the very minimum on an annual basis in all athletes. If levels are deficient or insufficient, athletes should supplement with vitamin D to help decrease the risk of injuries and illness while possibly improving performance.

CHAPTER 10

Iron

One of the most common questions I hear from female athletes transitioning to a plant-based or plant-forward diet is, "How do I make sure I'm getting enough iron?" It is a valid concern: iron deficiency is the most common nutritional deficiency worldwide and one of the most common concerns for women of childbearing age. Deficiency in iron can occur through increased needs (mainly, during menstruation), insufficient iron intake, or decreased absorption. Another common misconception is that you will not be able to get enough iron from plants. However, iron deficiency anemia does not occur in vegans and plant-based eaters any more than meat eaters.

This could be for several reasons:

1. Plant-based foods are very rich in iron.

2. Plant-based foods are also very rich in vitamin C and carotenoids, which can increase iron absorption five-fold and three-fold, respectively.

3. Vegans and plant-based eaters tend to have lower iron stores (but still within normal range) compared to meat eaters and lower stores can enhance the absorption and decrease the excretion of iron.

Iron: The Basics

Iron is a mineral that the body needs to support oxygenation throughout the body, muscle metabolism, healthy connective tissue, and growth and development. It is an essential component of hemoglobin, a protein in red blood cells that is responsible for carrying oxygen from the lungs throughout the body for use in the tissues. As a component of myoglobin (another protein that provides oxygen) iron supports muscle metabolism and healthy connective tissue. Iron is also necessary for physical growth, neurological development, cellular functioning, and synthesis of some hormones.

How Much Iron?

The Recommended Dietary Allowance (RDA) for all age groups of men and post-menopausal women is 8 milligrams a day; the RDA for premenopausal women is 18 milligrams a day.

However, the Food and Nutrition Board suggests that vegetarian and vegan iron needs may be higher than the RDA because **non-heme iron** (the type of iron found in plant-based foods) is not absorbed as well as **heme iron** (the type of iron found in animal tissue) due to phytates present in plant foods. For this reason, they suggest that vegetarians and vegans could require as much as 1.8 times more iron than those who eat meat.

However, these guidelines do not factor the effect of vitamin C, carotenoids, and allium vegetables on iron's absorbability or the fact that lower iron stores found in plant-based eaters may enhance iron absorption. That said, depending on the individual, some (including women with heavy menstruation and athletes) may indeed need more iron than what is recommended. If you suspect that you are not receiving enough and have symptoms of iron deficiency such as fatigue, easily bruising, or hair loss, then have your iron levels checked to determine your individual needs.

RECOMMENDED DAILY AMOUNT OF IRON		
Age	Male	Female
14–18 years	11 mg	15 mg
19–50 years	8 mg	18 mg
51+ years	8 mg	8 mg

Adequate Intake (AI) from https://ods.od.nih.gov/factsheets/Iron-HealthProfessional/

Increasing Iron Absorption

The primary plant-based culprit interfering with iron absorption is **phytic acid** (also known as phytates). While many plants are abundant in iron, their iron absorption can vary depending on the phytic acid content (in the same way oxalates can bind calcium, as we discussed in Chapter 8).

Let's first clear up any misconceptions—phytic acid is *not* a bad thing. It is actually an antioxidant that has been associated with a lower risk of cancer. It is naturally abundant in whole grains, legumes, nuts, and seeds. The key is to minimize its effect on binding to minerals like iron and zinc so that their absorption is maximized, which may be something that you are already doing.

There are several ways to minimize phytic acid binding to iron and maximize iron absorption:

1. Consume foods high in vitamin C (tomatoes, oranges, peppers, potatoes, broccoli) with iron-rich foods.
2. Cook iron-rich foods with allium vegetables (garlic, onions, shallots).
3. Consume iron-rich foods with foods rich in carotenoids (carrots, sweet potatoes, leafy greens).
4. Consume iron-rich fermented foods (for example, iron in fermented sourdough is better absorbed than iron in traditional bread).

Vitamin C

Consuming foods high in vitamin C along with plant-based iron-rich foods can increase iron absorption five-fold. Good sources of iron include beans, lentils, spinach, bok choy, tofu, tempeh, quinoa, tahini, prunes, peas, and more. Good sources of vitamin C include broccoli, tomatoes, citrus, avocados, red peppers, strawberries, guava, and more.

Examples of high iron and high vitamin C combinations include tacos with black beans and salsa, oatmeal and blueberries, lentils and sweet potatoes, or a spinach salad with orange slices.

Beta Carotene

Studies have shown that **carotenoids** like beta carotene, the plant-based version of vitamin A, can increase iron absorption by up to three times.

Carotenoids are a large group of compounds that give orange, yellow and red plants their color. There are more than 600 types of carotenoids and include some with which you may be familiar: beta carotene, lycopene, zeaxanthin, and lutein. Leafy greens are also high in carotenoids. Foods high in carotenoids include sweet potatoes, yams, leafy greens, watermelon, cantaloupe, bell peppers, tomatoes, carrots, mangoes and oranges.

Allium Vegetables

Do you cook with onion and garlic? Not only do these allium vegetables provide tons of flavor and nutrition, but they also may increase iron's absorption in plants by seven times! Add garlic and onion to soups and stews that include legumes, use them in stir fries with spinach, add minced garlic to your cooking water when cooking quinoa to give it flavor and to increase iron absorption. Allium vegetables include garlic, red onion, white onion, yellow onion, green onion, and scallions.

Finally, here are some additional tips for getting enough iron on a plant-based diet:

- Include organic soy foods in your diet, such as tempeh and tofu. The iron in soybeans is in a different form than other plant foods and does not appear to be affected as much by phytic acid.

- Consider getting some of your grains from whole grain bread, as the leavening process makes iron more absorbable.

- Space iron-rich foods throughout the day to potentially increase absorption.

- Avoid drinking coffee, tea or red wine when consuming high iron meals as they can inhibit iron absorption. Try to allow for 2 hours before or after eating meals rich in iron.

- Take calcium supplements separately from an iron-rich meal as calcium can impair absorption.

- Try soaking or fermentation. Phytates in some iron-rich plant-based foods decrease the bioavailability but soaking can help to increase absorption and decrease phytates. For example, soak beans overnight before cooking.

IRON CONTENT IN FOODS		
Food	**Serving Size**	**Iron Content**
Almonds	¼ cup	1.3 mg
Bagel, enriched	1 medium	3.8 mg
Black beans, cooked	1 cup	3.6 mg
Black eyed peas, cooked	1 cup	4.3 mg
Blackstrap molasses	2 tablespoons	7.2 mg
Broccoli, cooked	1 cup	1.0 mg
Chickpeas, cooked	1 cup	4.7 mg
Dark Chocolate, 45–69% cacao	3 ounces	7.0 mg
Kale, cooked	1 cup	1.0 mg
Kidney beans, cooked	1 cup	5.2 mg
Lentils, cooked	1 cup	6.6 mg
Lima beans, cooked	1 cup	4.5 mg
Millet, cooked	1 cup	1.1 mg
Natto (fermented soybean)	1 cup	15 mg
Pinto beans, cooked	1 cup	3.6 mg
Sesame seeds	2 tablespoons	1.2 mg
Soybeans, cooked	1 cup	4.5 mg
Spinach, cooked	1 cup	6.4 mg
Sunflower seeds	¼ cup	1.2 mg
Swiss chard, cooked	1 cup	4.0 mg
Tempeh	1 cup	4.5 mg
Tofu	½ cup	6.6 mg
Tomato juice	8 ounces	1.0 mg

Turnip greens, cooked	1 cup	1.2 mg
Veggie hot dog, iron-fortified	1 hot dog	3.6 mg
Watermelon	1/8 medium	1.4 mg

IRON AND VITAMIN C FOODS			
Food	Serving Size	Iron Content	Vitamin C Content
Tofu and Cooked Broccoli	½ cup, 1 cup	6.6 mg	102 mg
Tempeh and Cooked Brussel sprouts	1 cup, 1 cup	4.5 mg	96 mg
Cooked Spinach and Potatoes	1 cup, 1 medium	6.4 mg	42 mg
Cooked Kale and Tomato sauce (soup)	1 cup, 8 ounces	1.0 mg	45 mg
Raw Spinach and orange slices (salad)	1 cup, 1 small	1.0 mg	51 mg
Lentils and tomato sauce (chili)	1 cup, 1 cup	6.6 mg	80 mg
Watermelon and strawberries (fruit salad)	1/8 medium, 1 cup	1.4 mg	85 mg
Black beans and bell peppers (fajitas)	1 cup, 1 medium	3.6 mg	70 mg
Dark chocolate and strawberries (dessert)	3 ounces, ½ cup	7.0 mg	42 mg
Oatmeal and blueberries	1 cup, 1 cup	13.9 mg	14 mg

Iron Supplementation

Iron supplements, just like most vitamin and mineral supplements, are not benign. They are useful in times when intake or body stores are low but may not be beneficial or needed daily for long periods of time. In fact, once iron stores are adequate, iron supplementation does not help and may even cause side effects and toxicity.

Iron deficiency treatment could include oral supplements, intramuscular or intra-venous injections, and dietary intervention. Although iron supplements and injections have shown improved iron status in athletes, these methods often cause side effects like abdominal discomfort, constipation and nausea and may present a risk of too much iron. **Optimizing iron intake and absorption through the diet is suggested**

as the first line of action and primary strategy to prevent iron deficiency in both female and male athletes.

Considering an iron supplement to enhance performance? Sorry to be the bearer of bad news, but iron supplementation does not improve performance in non-depleted individuals. Only proper training will improve overall maximal performance. So, iron supplementation, whether pharmacologic or dietary, should be aimed at maintaining adequate iron stores and availability, not trying to exceed the body's demands.

Iron: The Bottom Line

Iron deficiency can impact oxidative capacity of muscle, protein synthesis, cognitive function, behavior, and body temperature regulation. Since athletes may be at higher risk of iron deficiency, it is important to have your healthcare provider check iron stores once or twice a year. Supplementation without checking stores is not recommended since excessive iron can also have negative implications. Optimizing iron intake and absorption through food first is always recommended.

CHAPTER 11

Vitamin B12

I f there is one nutrient to consider supplementing from day one of eating vegan or vegetarian, it is vitamin B12. It's especially important for athletes because it supports energy metabolism and oxygen transporting red blood cells. You do not need much B12, but what you do need plays a big role in many body functions. Chronic, severe deficiency of vitamin B12 can lead to anemia, dementia, and nerve damage. Becoming deficient in B12 can take up to a year and often without symptoms so my personal recommendation is for anyone moving toward a plant-based diet to start taking B12.

Vitamin B12: The Basics

Of all the known vitamins, B12 is the largest, with the most complex structure. It is water-soluble, meaning that your body uses what it needs and excretes the rest in your urine. (Some people can store the vitamin for up to four years; however, storage is not a reliable tactic to prevent deficiency.)

In its center is a single atom of cobalt, which is why B12 supplements are also known as cobalamins. Your body requires B12 to synthesize DNA, form red blood cells, maintain healthy bones, and keep your brain and nerves functioning. B12 is also essential for folate (another B vitamin) metabolism. Folate is important for reproduction and preventing anemia.

Vitamin B12 Deficiency

B12 can be tricky because even with adequate intake, absorption depends on other physiological factors. **Two steps are required for the body to absorb vitamin B12 from food.** First, hydrochloric acid in the stomach separates vitamin B12 from the protein in food. After this, vitamin B12 combines with intrinsic factor, a protein made by the stomach. Intrinsic factor helps your intestines absorb B12.

Pernicious anemia is an autoimmune disorder in people who cannot make intrinsic factor. As a result, they have trouble absorbing vitamin B12 from all foods and dietary supplements. It is a rare condition, with a prevalence of 0.1 percent in the general population and 1.9 percent in people who are older than 60 years, according to one study. That said, up to 50 percent of anemia from B12 deficiency in adults is caused by pernicious anemia, which is typically treated with B12 shots or high doses of an oral supplement. If you do not get enough vitamin B12, either because of inadequate intake or poor absorption, you are at risk of a B12 deficiency.

Common symptoms of B12 deficiency include fatigue, weakness, constipation, loss of appetite, weight loss, tingling of hands and feet, sore mouth or tongue, difficulty balancing, confusion, and poor memory.

Deficiency of B12 can also cause depression, neurological disorders, cardiovascular disease, neural tube defects, and has also been linked to dementia and breast cancer.

Interestingly, vitamin B12 also has antioxidant properties and can protect your cells from damage caused by free radicals and possibly reduce the risk of cancer.

Important for everyone, and especially athletes, Vitamin B12 ensures you have enough red blood cells in circulation, supporting oxygen availability throughout your body. It may also improve athletic performance. A 2020 study examined 1,131 blood samples collected from 243 track and field athletes over six years and compared the results to athletic performance. The researchers found that the ideal athletic performance was achieved when blood levels of B12 were in the range of 400–700 pg/mL (picograms per milliliter or one trillionth of a gram for those of you who are dying to know). Another study looking at iron, folate and B12 status of male and female Ethiopian professional runners found that increases in performance were associated with higher red blood cell counts, supported by normal iron, folate and B12 stores.

Vitamin B12 Supplementation

The best way to know if your B12 levels are normal is through a urine or blood test to determine your levels of methylmalonic acid (MMA). MMA is a substance created when your body digests protein, with B12 controlling how much MMA you make. High MMA indicates B12 deficiency.

You can also have serum B12 checked, but it is considered less reliable than MMA. A serum B12 above 400 pg/mL is considered optimal. Patients with B12 levels between 200 and 300 pg/mL are considered borderline. Patients with B12 levels below 200 pg/mL are considered deficient. Levels between 200 and 400 pg/mL are enough to prevent deficiency but still not optimal.

Vitamin B12 deficiency can affect anyone, but some groups of people that are at higher risk. While there is little research on B12 status in athletes, some athletes may experience the common causes of B12 deficiency. The most common cause of B12 deficiency is malabsorption, often seen in conditions like irritable bowel disease, Celiac disease, or bacterial overgrowth in the small intestine. The elderly population is more likely to have B12 deficiency, which could be related to poor dietary intake, decreased levels of hydrochloric acid, pernicious anemia and malabsorption syndromes. Finally, people who follow an exclusively plant-based or vegan diet are at risk of deficiency if they do not optimize their meal plan or supplement with vitamin B12.

The recommendation for B12 is 2.4 mcg for children over 14 years and all adult women and men.

If you prefer to get your nutrients from whole foods, then you might be interested in knowing which plant-based foods contain B12 so that you can at least try to include them in your diet. Plant-based whole food sources include algae, seaweed, some mushrooms, and some fermented foods (tempeh, kimchi, sauerkraut, and miso). However, many of these plants contain inactive B12 compounds that are similar to vitamin B12 but don't have any vitamin activity. Reliable sources of vitamin B12 for vegans include B12 foods fortified with this nutrient like plant-based milk and nutritional yeast.

If you follow a plant-based diet, it is important to consider a B12 supplement to meet your needs.

B12 Supplements

You can find two types of B12 supplements on the market. **The two forms of B12 include cyanocobalamin and methylcobalamin.** Cyanocobalamin is the inactive form of B12. Your body converts it into the two active forms, methylcobalamin or adenosylcobalamin, both of which have different functions.

Some studies indicate that cyanocobalamin may be better absorbed. Others suggest that cyanocobalamin is the best choice for most people because it is the least expensive, most stable form, it has been well studied and proven to increase vitamin B12 status. That said, it is synthetically made and is attached to a cyanide molecule (hence, the name "cyano" in cyanocobalamin). The quantity of cyanide is so low that it will not do damage and will be excreted in the urine, but, for some, that might be a concern.

Methylcobalamin is the natural form of B12 (the kind found in food sources). Some studies have found that, compared to methylcobalamin, more cyanocobalamin is excreted through urine, suggesting that methylcobalamin may be retained better.

Overall, available research around vitamin B12 suggests that the differences in the bioavailability between the two forms is probably not enough to suggest one over the other. Instead, factors that affect the absorption of vitamin B12, like age and individual absorption issues, may be more influential than the form of the supplement itself.

How much vitamin B12 should you take in the form of a supplement? **It is best to get your levels tested to determine your baseline and adjust dosages accordingly.** B12 absorption, even from a supplement, is very low. If you are trying to maximize absorption it might be best to split your dose 2–3 times throughout the day.

Vitamin B12: The Bottom Line

Again, if you are a whole foods purist and want to optimize B12 through diet then consider eating three to four servings a day of food fortified with 2 to 3.5 mcg of B12 each. If you are not consuming B12 fortified foods, then you definitely want to take a supplement. Depending on your B12 stores, consider taking 25 to 250 mcg of B12 in the form of cobalamin or methylcobalamin daily or 1000 to 2000 mcg once or twice a week. Both liquid for sublingual supplementation or a capsule should both be equally effective.

CHAPTER 12

Iodine

Despite being one of the first nutrients recognized as essential to humans, two billion people worldwide are deficient in iodine.

Iodine: The Basics

Naturally found in soil and sea water, iodine is not made by your body, and therefore needs to be a part of your diet. **Iodine is essential for the synthesis of thyroid hormones, which play an essential role in metabolism, enzyme activity, and proper bone and brain development during pregnancy and infancy.** Obtaining sufficient iodine is important for everyone, especially for women, infants, and children. Lack of iodine can also cause goiter, which is an enlargement of the thyroid gland. When there is insufficient iodine, your thyroid gland enlarges in effort to work harder to make thyroid hormones.

Iodine Deficiency

For those who follow a vegan diet or eat mostly plant-based, unless you are consciously using iodized salt daily, or eating sea vegetables often, you might not be getting enough iodine in your diet. Foods that are highest in iodine include dairy, eggs, fish, and sea vegetables (like seaweed, kelp, dulse, and nori). Salty packaged soups and restaurant foods typically contain regular table salt (sodium and chloride) that is not fortified with iodine since table salt is less expensive to use than iodized salt. Those fancy salts that claim to be loaded with natural minerals (looking at you, sea salt, pink Himalayan salt, and Celtic salt) are also not reliable sources of iodine.

Vegans and plant-based enthusiasts tend to eat a lot of cruciferous vegetables, which are high in goitrogens. **Goitrogens** are substances that can be naturally occurring in foods and can disrupt the production of thyroid hormones by interfering with iodine uptake in the thyroid gland. This can trigger the pituitary gland to release **thyroid stimulating hormone (TSH)**, which then stimulates thyroid tissue growth and may possibly lead to goiter in the absence of sufficient iodine. Foods high in goitrogens include soy-based products, broccoli, kale and flaxseed. The trick is not to avoid these foods, but to get enough iodine.

Vegan Sources of Iodine

Seaweed can be a decent source of iodine, but the amount varies and may sometimes contain too much. Some kelp contains iodine that far exceeds the recommended amount. Wakame, nori, and arame might be safer choices. Since sea vegetables can sometimes absorb heavy metals (mercury and arsenic) in the same way they efficiently absorb minerals (iodine, calcium and iron), look for organic sources and sea vegetables harvested from brands that do third-party testing for heavy metals. The amount of iodine in just ¼ teaspoon of iodized salt is 71 mcg, almost half of daily needs. Multivitamins are also an option, which typically contain the recommended 150 mcg.

How Much Iodine?

The Dietary Reference Intake for Iodine is 150 mcg a day for adults. More is needed during pregnancy (220 mcg per day) to assist with fetal development. As with any nutrient, more is not better. (I think you got this message by now.) The upper tolerable limit for iodine in adults is 1100 mcg a day.

Iodine: The Bottom Line

So, what is a vegan to do? First, please continue to eat organic soy products and cruciferous veggies. They are too good for you to give up for a finicky little mineral. Just make sure you use iodized salt in cooking, consume organic sea vegetables during the week or take a multivitamin that includes iodine. If you incorporate one of these tactics, then you should be receiving adequate amounts of the mineral.

CHAPTER 13

Magnesium

While calcium, iron and B12 might be the nutrients of highest concern to many swapping plants for dairy and meat, there is another nutrient that should be on the plant-based athlete's radar: **magnesium**. Magnesium deficiency is so common that it has been called a public health crisis. Even though this mineral is naturally found in many foods and is the fourth most abundant mineral in our body, between 10–30 percent of people worldwide and 50 percent of Americans appear to be not getting enough for optimal health.

Similar to iron deficiency, magnesium deficiency is not just a vegan or vegetarian issue. **It is actually not difficult to meet magnesium needs when you are eating a whole plant-based food diet, since magnesium is mostly found in plants.** The reason so many are not getting enough magnesium in their diet is because most people in the United States consume the standard American diet (SAD) which is high in processed packaged foods and lacking in plant-based nutrition.

Magnesium: The Basics

Magnesium is involved in more than 300 enzyme systems that regulate a variety of biochemical reactions in the body, including protein synthesis, muscle and nerve function, blood glucose control, and blood pressure regulation. Magnesium is required for energy production and the breakdown of glucose for energy.

Magnesium is also essential for the conversion of muscle glycogen to glucose, your body's fuel during intense exercise, as it is needed to generate ATP (adenosine triphosphate). Without sufficient magnesium, lactic acid build-up, resulting in muscle soreness and fatigue. It is also key in protein synthesis, aiding in recovery. As you can see, magnesium plays a key role in performance, training goals, recovery, and bone health. In fact, every cell in your body contains it and needs it to function!

Magnesium and Athletic Performance

There are several ways in which magnesium plays an important role in athletic performance:

- Energy release: Helps convert food into energy
- Protein synthesis: Helps create new proteins from amino acids
- Gene maintenance: Helps create and repair DNA and RNA
- Electrolyte balance: Helps to maintain electrolyte balance
- Muscle movements: Assists with contraction and relaxation of muscles
- Nervous system regulation: Helps regulate neurotransmitters, which send messages throughout your brain and nervous system

Research shows that athletes participating in strenuous exercise may require 10–20 percent more magnesium than the general population due to sweat and urinary losses. Dietary surveys show that male athletes consume less than 260 mg magnesium per day and female athletes consume less than 220 mg magnesium per day. There's also evidence showing that marginal magnesium deficiency impairs exercise performance, increases oxidative stress (a consequence of strenuous exercise) and increases blood pressure.

While magnesium supplementation or increased intake of magnesium-rich foods can improve performance in magnesium deficient athletes, magnesium supplementation on top of adequate magnesium intake and stores is controversial. One of the limiting factors is that it is challenging to determine magnesium levels in an individual. The general consensus appears to be that magnesium supplementation has a greater effect when dietary magnesium intake is habitually low.

Overall, if magnesium has not been on your radar, athletes, then it is time to check your dietary magnesium intake. Are you getting enough? If you are experiencing fatigue, poor recovery, or muscle soreness, now would be a good time to include more leafy greens, whole grains, legumes, nuts and seeds into your diet as lack of magnesium could be your issue. Replacing processed foods with whole foods can be one step toward adequate magnesium intake. For example, instead of boxed mac n cheese (zero magnesium), make legume mac n cheese with chickpea macaroni, cashew cheese and broccoli, which has 115 mg magnesium per serving (see recipe on page 190).

How Much Magnesium?

So how much magnesium should you be aiming for? The Recommended Dietary Allowances (RDA) for magnesium varies with age:

- Boys 14–18 years: 410 mg
- Girls 14–18 years: 360 mg
- Men 19+ years: 400–420 mg
- Women 19+ years: 310–320 mg

Vegan Sources of Magnesium

The single most important way to consume magnesium is through your diet. I have good news, plant-based enthusiasts! The foods high in magnesium are also high in many other nutrients that your body needs to thrive. There is little magnesium in meat, dairy, and eggs. Foods high in magnesium include nuts, seeds, soy milk, tofu, tempeh, avocado, beets, beans, bananas, cauliflower, teff, amaranth and dark chocolate.

There is no need to count magnesium to ensure you are getting enough, unless you suspect that you are not and want to check yourself by writing down what you eat and drink in a day and calculate the magnesium content in your diet (cronometer.com is a great resource for this). **By simply eating a variety of whole plant-based foods, you can receive enough magnesium.** Similar to iron, phytic acid can impair magnesium absorption. By following the same steps to reduce phytic acids (consuming foods high in vitamin C, carotenes, and allium vegetables) with magnesium-rich foods helps to increase magnesium absorption. Again, since many plant-based foods are already rich in vitamin C and carotenoids, it is pretty simple to implement this practice.

For more information about the magnesium content of specific plant-based foods beneficial to an athlete's diet, see page 221 under Tables and References at the back of this book.

Magnesium: The Bottom Line

Since magnesium is abundant in plant-based foods, I recommend getting your magnesium through whole foods. However, if you suspect that you are not getting enough you can complement the magnesium in your diet with a supplement and, again, not exceeding 400 mg a day.

CHAPTER 14

Zinc

Zinc is the second most abundant mineral in our body, right after iron. We do not make it; therefore, it's essential. **Zinc is needed for more than 50 different enzyme reactions in the body, which means that it's pretty important for a lot of physiological processes.** It supports the immune system, plays a role in wound healing, assists with metabolism and is important for growth in children.

While it is abundant in foods, it's not uncommon for people to get suboptimal amounts of zinc, which can affect the immune system, sense of taste and smell, carbohydrates metabolism and DNA synthesis. Many studies show that vegans have zinc intakes similar to that of omnivores, while others show that zinc intake may be insufficient in vegans due to phytates present which can bind zinc in plant-based foods, similar to iron. That said, zinc deficiency is rare in vegans and the general population of the United States. It's worth mentioning here because of its importance in supporting immune health and many enzyme reactions and because those eating plant-based may need more compared to meat eaters.

How Much Zinc?

The amount of zinc you need each day depends on your age. Average daily recommended amounts for different ages are listed below in milligrams (mg):

DAILY RECOMMENDED AMOUNT OF ZINC	
Life Stage	**Recommended Amount (mg)**
Teens 14–18 years (boys)	11 mg
Teens 14–18 years (girls)	9 mg
Adults (men)	11 mg
Adults (women)	8 mg

Similar to iron, **phytates** can bind zinc in foods. For that reason, it has been suggested that vegans or those eating all plant-based may need up to 50 percent more than the RDA for zinc. Using that rule of thumb, men eating an all plant-based diet would need 16.5 mg zinc a day and women would need 12 mg a day, which is not difficult to get when you're consuming nutrient-dense plant-based foods. Other groups at risk for decreased zinc absorption include individuals with gastrointestinal disorders as much of zinc absorption is regulated in the intestine.

Vegan Sources of Zinc

Adding zinc daily is not difficult when you consider that the following food servings have 1 mg of zinc:

- 1 tablespoon of nuts, seeds, or nut/seed butters
- ¼ to ½ cup cooked beans
- 1 tablespoon wheat germ
- 1 cup cooked whole grains
- 3 ounces tofu
- 2 slices of bread
- 2 cups cooked leafy green vegetables

If you consume plant-based meats, check their nutrition labels since some of these are fairly high in zinc. Fortified cereals are also very high in their zinc content. When in doubt, add pumpkin seeds. This is my personal go-to food since it's easy to sprinkle on salads, add to granola or cereal, add to muffins and baked goods, or simply snack on a handful during the day. Just ¼ cup of pumpkin seeds has 2.2 mg zinc.

Finally, some of the same practices that allow iron to be more readily absorbed may also help with zinc absorption such as choosing fermented foods like sourdough bread and tempeh, soaking nuts, seeds, and legumes, and avoiding coffee and tea with meals.

Zinc Supplementation

Upper tolerable limit for zinc is 40 mg a day because it can compete with copper, another essential mineral. Supplements should only be taken for short periods of time as they can cause anemia if taken too long. Also, zinc supplementation can cause nausea and flu-like symptoms when taken in high amounts.

Zinc: The Bottom Line

Eating a variety of plant-based foods should ensure that you are getting plenty of zinc. However, if you suspect you are not, then check your intake (cronometer.com to the rescue once again!) and supplement as needed, but only short term.

CHAPTER 15

Selenium

Okay, last micronutrient, not of all time, but at least the last I wanted to mention that is very important for hormones, metabolism, immunity and protection from oxidative damage. Introducing...selenium! This trace element is naturally present in soil but because soil differs around the world, the final quantities of selenium can vary in plant-based foods, leaving some folks with inadequate intake.

Selenium: The Basics

Since selenium acts as an antioxidant, it can reduce free radicals and the oxidative stress they pose on the body leading to diseases like heart disease, Alzheimer's disease, and cancer. **Selenium also supports immune function and, in research, has been shown to enhance immunity and fight viral infections.** Research has suggested that those with asthma have lower serum levels of selenium and adequate intakes of this mineral may help reduce asthma-related symptoms.

Selenium is also essential for an optimal functioning thyroid. Fun fact: thyroid tissue contains more selenium than any other organ in the body! The thyroid gland is important since it regulates metabolism and controls growth and development. One observational study looked at 6,000 people from China (where selenium intake can be suboptimal due to low selenium in the soil) and found that low serum selenium levels were associated with an increased risk of autoimmune thyroiditis and hypothyroidism. Another review concluded that taking selenium supplements daily for three months led to improvement in mood and well-being in those with hypothyroidism. That said, more research is needed before selenium supplementation is recommended in hypo-thyroidism as excessive selenium can be detrimental as well (surprise!).

Selenium Needs for Athletes

Exhaustive physical exercise can create oxidant damage by promoting free radical production in muscle, liver, heart and lung tissue. Because selenium plays a role in antioxidant defense, researchers have investigated whether or not selenium supplementation can improve performance and recovery. One study looked at serum and urinary selenium levels in long distance runners from Spain compared to sedentary individuals and found that serum selenium concentrations were lower in the runners, suggesting that physical activity may increase the need for selenium.

However, a 2020 meta-analysis, reviewing six solid studies, looked at selenium supplementation in athletes and found that selenium supplementation did not improve performance, exercise adaptation or antioxidants effects. In addition, supplementation showed a negative effect on mitochondria (the energy powerhouse of our cells) in chronic and acute exercise. They concluded that the use of selenium supplementation has no benefits on aerobic or anaerobic athletic performance, but it may prevent selenium deficiencies among athletes with high-intensity and high-volume training. **Like many of the micronutrients, it is important to optimize selenium through food.** The recommendation for selenium is 55 mcg a day for adult males and females and children over 14 years of age.

While selenium toxicity is rare, it is important to not to exceed the tolerable upper limit of 400 mcg per day. Selenium toxicity has been reported.

Vegan Sources of Selenium

While it is tough to say exactly how much selenium you're getting from food since the amount can vary so much depending on the soil, there are some plant-based foods that are solid sources of selenium. The most well-known source of selenium in the plant kingdom is Brazil nuts. By simply eating one or two Brazil nuts a day can help you meet your selenium needs since each nut contains 175 percent or more of the RDA for selenium as well as other essential micronutrients like zinc, copper, and magnesium (again, this depends on the soil in which it's grown, but on average, one nut a day can help you meet your needs). A bonus is that the phytonutrients in tree nuts, including Brazil nuts, have been associated with reduced inflammation. Brazil nuts contain several nutrients that act as antioxidants, including selenium, vitamin E and phytonutrients, or phenols, like gallic acid and ellagic acid, all of which have been shown to reduce inflammation and protect your body from oxidative stress.

Snacking on a few Brazil nuts a day can be the perfect way to enjoy a tasty and crunchy snack while getting your daily intake of selenium. Allergic to nuts? Other sources of selenium include mushrooms, amaranth, whole grain bread, brown rice, pinto beans, tofu, chia seeds, and sunflower seeds.

Selenium: The Bottom Line

Getting sufficient selenium through foods is important for athletic performance and recovery. Eat one or two Brazil nuts daily or consume a variety of plant-based foods that contain selenium to get your daily intake of selenium.

VEGAN
ATHLETE FOCUS
TOPICS

CHAPTER 16

Bone Health

Bones are a bit complicated. Bone growth, strength and maintenance go beyond getting enough calcium and vitamin D. Athletes should pay special attention to bone health in order to reduce the risk of injury short term and ensure strong bones long term, avoiding osteopenia and osteoporosis later in life. Modifying training loads by reducing training intensity or duration could prevent injury, however, for some coaches and athletes this is not an option. Therefore, it is important to support training loads by optimizing nutrition.

Bone Health and Athletes

Around 90 percent of bone mass is attained during early adulthood (early twenties), with the peak amount of bone mass (also called bone mineral density or BMD) forming at around 30 years of age. It is important to implement practices that support BMD early in life to set yourself up for osteopenia and osteoporosis prevention later in life.

For most athletes, the immediate concern is avoiding injury, which causes an interruption in training. **When bone health is suboptimal (meaning bone mass and bone strength cannot support training), stress fractures can occur.** While studies on athletes specifically are limited, general population studies show that there are many reasons why bone mass and bone strength may not be optimal. Groups that may be at more risk for low BMD include endurance runners, swimmers and cyclists, compared to strength athletes or rugby players. Those in sports that encourage low body weight and smaller frames such as dancers, gymnasts, and jockeys are also at higher risk for low BMD.

Caloric intake, including carbohydrates, protein, and fat intake can all play a part in bone formation and preventing bone loss. Micronutrient intake such as calcium, vitamin D, magnesium and, more recently of focus, vitamin K2, all play a role. Calcium and sodium losses through sweat may also contribute to mineral loss and suboptimal bone health in athletes. All of these factors can affect hormones, which regulate bone health. It's not simple, but we will talk about ways to optimize bone health whether you are in your early 20's and need to support bone growth or if you are at a stage where you need to prevent bone loss.

Nutrition and Bone Health

To demonstrate the complexity of bone health, can you guess how many vitamins and minerals are involved with supporting bone mass and strength? You know of three— calcium, vitamin D and magnesium—but it might surprise you to learn there are at least 18 nutrients involved in bone health. There are even more that assist calcium with actually getting into the bone, such as vitamin K2. Specific nutrients that play a role in bone health include boron, B vitamins, iron, vitamin A, copper, manganese, phosphorus, potassium, silica, vitamin C, zinc, phytonutrients, protein, and omega 3 fatty acids.

Receiving adequate calories may be the single most important first step in supporting bone formation and preventing bone loss as caloric intake from adequate carbohydrates, protein, and fat supports hormones that regulate bone turnover. Studies show that decreased bone formation can occur when calories do not support training loads. If low caloric intake is maintained over a period of time, then it could potentially lead to osteopenia or osteoporosis and fractures that will clearly impact performance.

Low carbohydrates, high protein and high fat diets are often promoted to help meet body composition goals. There are many reasons why I do not recommend a low-carb diet for the general population (see chapter on carbs if you would like another primer) and especially for athletes. One of these reasons is that it may attenuate bone loss. Some research shows that low carbohydrates diets could negatively affect bone health, especially when followed alongside a high-fat diet.

It has also been theorized that diets high in animal protein, which is acidic, may cause more calcium to leach from the bone to balance the acidity since calcium is alkaline. Scientists suggested that this would lead to the breakdown of bone tissue to release calcium, with excess calcium being excreted in the urine. However, that theory has been unfounded and more recent evidence shows that adequate protein, whether it comes from animals or plants, supports bone health. What is most important is that athletes consume sufficient protein as well as sufficient calcium to support bone formation and turnover.

That said, a plant-based diet can include many of the nutrients to support strong bones. **Whole plant-based foods are brimming with vitamins C, K, antioxidants and phytonutrients — all of which have shown to promote healthy bones.** In particular, phytonutrients called isoflavones, found in soy, beans, and peas, have been shown to increase bone mineral density by stimulating bone formation and decreasing bone resorption. Adequately planned whole food plant-based diets can also supply plenty of protein and calcium. Bone-supporting nutrients that are found in some plants, but may need to be supplemented include B12, vitamin D, and omega 3's. The addition of antioxidants and phytonutrients in plants, which are minimal or obsolete in animal products, may position plants as a superior source to meat when it comes to bone health.

Vitamin A vs Beta Carotene

It is also worth mentioning the role of vitamin A in bone health. Adequate vitamin A can support bone growth while too much vitamin A has been shown to be detrimental to bone health. Vitamin A is only found in animal products. Plant-based foods contain beta carotene, a phytonutrient that is converted to vitamin A in the body. Some studies show that beta carotene can more effectively contribute to bone health without the detrimental effects as seen with direct vitamin A intake from animal-based foods, which may be detrimental to bone health. (Another win for plants!)

Vitamin K1 and K2

Another essential vitamin that is important to mention is vitamin K. With emerging research, scientists are recognizing that vitamin K1 and vitamin K2 each have unique roles in the body, but both may play a role in bone health. Vitamin K1 is essential for blood clotting and vitamin K2 is essential for bone and heart health. Vitamin K1 (phylloquinone) can be easily obtained from a plant-based diet through cruciferous veggies, asparagus, peas, parsley, and leafy greens. Vitamin K2 (menaquinone) is made from human and animal gut bacteria.

Moderate amounts of K2 are found in fermented foods like kimchi, fermented kraut, tempeh and natto. It is also found in animal products such as butter, egg yolks, and organ meats. Gut bacteria may be able to convert some K1 to K2 but there are so many individual variables that it is not a reliable source of K2. Vitamin K2 helps with regulating calcium balance. This is important because calcium buildup can accumulate in the arteries causing calcification. **The role of vitamin K2 is to lead calcium into the bones, which not only supports bone health, but prevents it from building up in the arteries.** This is why you may see vitamin K in bone-specific supplements that include calcium and vitamin D.

The RDA for vitamin K1 is 90 micrograms a day for women and 120 micrograms a day for men. Plant-based foods rich in vitamin K1 include leafy greens, broccoli, Brussels sprouts, parsley, chia seeds, and edamame.

What about vitamin K2? Unfortunately, even though it is clear that K2 plays an important role in bone health, there is not yet a concrete recommendation for it. Based on certain studies, some scientists are suggesting 10–40 micrograms per day of K2.

While the amount of K2 in fermented foods can vary, consuming some sort of fermented foods daily may help directly deliver K2 and it may also promote healthy bacteria, which could possibly lead to making K2 in your gut. The exact amount you would be receiving is unknown. If your bones are healthy, you are getting enough calcium, vitamin D, calories (including a balance of carbohydrates, protein and fat), and a variety of plant-based foods, including some fermented foods, I do not believe there is a need to supplement with vitamin K2. However, if you're taking a calcium supplement, you may want to look for a supplement that also includes 10-40 micrograms of vitamin K2.

DERMAL LOSSES FROM SWEAT

Many endurance athletes fall into the category of **"heavy sweater,"** those wearing heavy uniforms and those just susceptible to lots of sweating. Endurance athletes are probably at most risk for suboptimal bone density due to their high caloric needs and when the activity is not weight bearing.

Calcium is lost through sweat during exercise, and the parathyroid hormone is released when low calcium is detected in the body. Parathyroid hormone triggers the bone to release calcium to maintain calcium homeostasis in the blood. The short-term calcium loss from bone may not be harmful but could result in bone loss long-term. Research has shown that ingesting calcium before intense endurance training may offset calcium dermal losses. So, if you're an elite endurance athlete with heavy sweat losses consuming calcium-rich foods before training is something to consider. A smoothie with leafy greens and fortified plant-based milk could do the trick.

Are Vegans at More Risk for Fractures?

There were big headlines in late 2020 that caught the public eye, "Vegans are at higher fracture risk compared to meat-eaters." The headline is a bit alarming, but let's break down the study. Researchers looked at 54,898 people living in the UK, 1,982 of whom were vegan, and found a greater risk of total and site-specific hip fractures in vegans compared to meat-eaters after an average follow-up of 17.6 years. The authors attributed some of the risk of fractures to low BMI and lower calcium and protein intakes among vegans.

The average protein intake was 12.9 percent and 13.5 percent of calories for vegan men and women, and 16 percent and 17.3 percent for meat-eaters. Calcium intake was 1,058 and 989 mg a day for meat-eating men and women, and 611 and 580 mg/day for vegan men and women, which is considerably lower and not meeting calcium needs. The low calcium intake in vegans may be a reflection of a processed vegan diet versus a diet rich in nutrient-dense plant-based foods. Supplement intake was unknown.

Twenty-nine percent of meat-eaters and 41 percent of vegans reported engaging in "moderate or high physical activity."

So, without knowing the vegan's specific intake of whole plant-based foods and whether or not they supplemented with vitamin D or vitamin K, it is tough to place all bets on this study. Other studies show that diets with adequate vegetable, fruit, mineral, and phytonutrient intake are linked to better bone health.

Bone Health: The Bottom Line

Overall recommendations for bone health include:

- Obtaining sufficient calcium, preferably from food (see Chapter 8 on calcium).
- Ensure you are getting adequate sunlight to produce vitamin D or taking supplements if warranted (See Chapter 9 on vitamin D).
- Eat plenty and a variety of plant-based foods rich in magnesium.
- Get the recommended amount of fiber plus fermented foods in your diet daily for vitamin K2 production.
- Eat enough calories and protein to support your needs.
- Avoid omitting any of the macronutrient groups (carbohydrates, protein, or fat) from your diet.
- Get 30 minutes of weight-bearing exercise daily to support bone health.
- Avoid excessive alcohol intake and smoking.
- Avoid excessive caffeine and salt.
- Avoid drinking soda.

Including a variety of plant protein sources like beans (including organic soy), seeds, nuts, and vegetables, provides adequate amounts of protein. This is important for bone health since certain essential amino acids facilitate collagen formation, an essential component of bone. Consuming 1–2 tablespoons daily of flax meal or chia seed can help you get omega 3's. Plant foods are naturally high in vitamin C, vitamin K, magnesium, carotenoids (plant-based vitamin A), potassium, copper, and B vitamins. Consuming a variety of colorful plants can ensure adequate intake of all these bone-supporting nutrients. Eating leafy greens daily, including nuts and seeds, organic soy (especially calcium treated tofu), and fortified plant-based milk can help you meet your calcium needs. What is left? Vitamins D and B12 will most likely need to be supplemented if you're not getting enough sun or consuming vitamin B12 fortified foods.

CHAPTER 17

Plant-Based Diets for Performance and Recovery

"Before going plant-based, I was thin and desired to be larger and stronger. I thought eating meat was the only way to increase muscle but the previous decades had shown otherwise. Once going plant-based, I was less fatigued following strength training and running while lifting more and running farther which enabled me to put on the mass I had been wanting. Cutting meat and dairy out while focusing primarily on healthful foods has enabled me to reach my initial goal and continue raising the bar with new ones. As a public health professional, living a healthful life and choosing plant-based foods has enabled me to walk the walk when promoting lifestyle choices which decrease the chance of chronic disease."

—**Chris,** vegan athlete and public health professional

One of the biggest benefits of whole food plant-based eating over a diet that includes meat, dairy, and processed foods is its effects on recovery and inflammation. The advantage that plants have over animal products are threefold:

1. Plants have an abundance of **phytonutrients**, plant compounds that are not made by animal products. These phytonutrients play a big role in fighting inflammation from tissue injury or outside toxins.

2. Plants have **fiber**, a nutrient not found in animal products. Fiber is the foundation to a healthy gut which results in less short- and long-term inflammation.

3. Plants have minimal to none of the compounds found in meat that result in **inflammation**, such as pollutants and hormones that are stored in the fat of animal products. Not only is the saturated fat itself inflammatory, but when the fat is broken down, the stored pollutants and pollutants are released into the body. (Enter phytonutrients to the rescue!)

Inflammation: The Basics

Inflammation is the body's natural protective response to a variety of stressors, including infection and injury.

Acute inflammation can occur when there is tissue damage due to trauma, pathogens (bacteria, viruses, or parasites), and other harmful compounds (environmental, alcohol, tobacco). When something damages your cells, your body reacts by releasing antibodies and proteins to the damaged area in order to resolve tissue damage by increasing blood flow and vessel permeability. The immediate signs are heat, pain, redness and swelling—all important for the body's repair and defense. This response can last for hours or days until this process clears the infection or repairs the damaged tissue.

Chronic inflammation happens when the response continues and leaves your body in a constant state of alert. It can occur with continued exposure to pathogens, continued trauma, and in some cases, when the body recognizes components of itself as foreign and attacks itself, i.e. autoimmune diseases.

For athletes, high-intensity exercises can create delayed onset muscle soreness (DOMS), which is a form of acute inflammation. Up to six hypothesized theories have been proposed for the mechanism of DOMS: lactic acid, muscle spasm, connective tissue damage, muscle damage, inflammation, and enzyme fluctuations. Scientists feel that it is a combination of two or more of these factors that create muscle soreness. Delayed onset muscle soreness typically occurs within the first 24 hours, peaks between 24 and 72 hours, and can last as long as 5–7 days after exercise. Delayed onset muscle soreness may lead to limited range of motion, affecting future training sessions. The effects of plant-based eating to expedite recovery are currently being investigated.

Inflammation and Athletes

Research shows that endurance athletes may have more advanced atherosclerosis and more myocardial damage compared with sedentary individuals, especially as they age. One study conducted in the UK showed that coronary plaques were found in 44 percent of middle-aged and older endurance athletes engaged in cycling or running, compared with 22 percent of sedentary subjects. Another study including 50 men who ran in at least 25 consecutive marathons in Twin Cities, MN, found the runners to have increased total plaque volume, calcified plaque volume, and non-calcified plaque volume, compared with 23 sedentary controls.

These studies show that well-trained athletes may be at risk for heart disease. What is unknown is whether these changes in aging athletes are a result of the athletic activity or the food that is consumed to fuel the activity since quick-acting carbohydrates and meat protein have traditionally been recommended. **This is a solid case for eating more plants as we know that the phytonutrients and fiber in plants can reduce the risk of heart disease.**

The Physicians Committee for Responsible Medicine (PCRM) reviewed several studies in 2019 looking at the ability of plant-based diets to reduce the risk of cardiovascular disease and how the diet affects performance. They concluded that plant-based eating may help to prevent the long-term inflammatory response, whether it is exercise or food induced atherosclerosis and myocardial damage by several ways:

1. **Lower body fat for performance advantage:** Lower body fat can increase the ability to use oxygen to fuel exercise. Studies show that athletes on a plant-based diet increase their VO2 max—the maximum amount of oxygen they can use during intense exercise—leading to better endurance. Endurance athletes on a plant-based diet often have lower body fat, which can give them a performance advantage.

2. **Increase blood flow and tissue oxygenation:** A low saturated fat diet (plants!) can improve blood flow, which can help more oxygen reach the muscles and ultimately improve athletic performance.

3. **Reduce oxidative stress and inflammation:** Plant-based eaters consume many more phytonutrients (often acting as antioxidants) which help to neutralize free radicals that lead to muscle fatigue, reduced athlete performance and impaired recovery.

4. **Lower risk of heart disease:** There's strong evidence that a plant-based diet keeps hearts strong by reversing plaque, bringing down blood pressure and cholesterol, and reducing weight.

5. **Omitting meat means less inflammation:** Consuming meat leads to inflammation, which can result in pain and impair athletic performance and recovery, whereas a plant-based diet can have the opposite effect.

The late and honorable, Susan Levin, RD, who was a board-certified specialist in sports dietetics and director of nutrition education for PCRM, states that these findings have relevance not just for professional or Olympic-level athletes. "Everyday athletes experience the same boost from a plant-based diet as gold medal Olympians, Super Bowl winners, and Wimbledon champions," Levin says. "The performance and recovery benefits provided by the fiber, carbohydrates, antioxidants, and other nutrients found in a plant-based diet are the same whether you're running a 5K or marathon."

How Phytonutrients Fight Inflammation

Plant-based foods contain more than 10,000 different disease-preventing compounds called phytonutrients (also known as phytochemicals, "phyto" meaning "plant"). Thankfully, scientists have been busy studying these nutrients therefore we know quite a bit about many of them. Anthocyanins in blueberries and other purple or blue-hued foods may help with cognition and memory. Lycopene, the red pigment in tomatoes, has been shown to fight prostate cancer. Gingerol in ginger has gone head-to-head with pain killers. Betalains in beets can increase blood flow.

These are just the beginning—there are so many more phytonutrients, and they have the ability to do so much when it comes to healing the body. Taking anthocyanins as an example, they have also been shown to lower LDL cholesterol, fight inflammation, and act as a prebiotic for healthy gut bacteria. Imagine what we could learn and uncover from studying the remaining nutrients?

Take dioxins as an example. **Dioxins are persistent organic (not in the good organic kind of way) pollutants, which means that they take a very long time to break down once they are in the environment.** Some of the highest levels of dioxins are found in meat, dairy, and fish. They are highly toxic and have been shown to cause cancer, disrupt hormones, and wreak havoc on the immune system. One study found that the phytonutrients in plant-based foods like fruits, vegetables, tea leaves and beans can block the effects of dioxins. Having phytonutrient levels in the bloodstream achieved by eating three apples a day or a tablespoon of red onion appears to cut dioxin toxicity *in half*.

However, the effect of plants only lasts for a few hours. So, in order to maintain the protection, you need to... eat plants at each meal! Also, since plants are naturally lower in fat compared to animal products, they are naturally lower in pollutants such as dioxins.

A SPECIAL NOD TO POLYPHENOLS

Polyphenols influence the taste and color of plants. When we eat them, they act like antioxidants by scavenging free radicals, dilating blood vessels by releasing nitric oxide, and fighting inflammation that results from intense exercise. Examples of foods packed with polyphenols include cloves, dark chocolate or cacao, berries, cherries, black beans, pecans, and green tea. You may have heard of flavonoids in dark chocolate, catechins in green tea, or anthocyanins in blueberries—these are all classified as polyphenols.

Some studies show that supplementation with approximately 300 mg polyphenols an hour prior to exercise may enhance endurance and repeated sprint performance, most likely due to improved muscle perfusion. Others show that supplementation with more than 1000 mg of polyphenols per day for 3 or more days before and following exercise may enhance recovery from exercise-induced damage. While there is growing evidence that short-term and long-term supplementation with fruit-derived polyphenols may enhance exercise performance, most likely due to their antioxidant and vascular effects, more research is needed. There is a larger body of evidence that suggests that consistent and long-term consumption of whole food polyphenols may enhance recovery from intensive exercise. Eat your plants to recover quickly and boost performance, friends!

There is a reason why numerous athletes are turning to a plant-based diet. It not only meets their nutritional needs and prevents lifestyle diseases, but also may give them an edge in performance and recovery.

CHAPTER 18

Sleep

"The first change that I noticed was better sleep, and it happened pretty quickly. I've never been a great sleeper, and this made significant improvements to my sleep quality. The second immediate change I experienced was how fast I recovered from workouts. Once I implemented plant-based eating, I never felt super worn down after consecutive days of hard sessions. Getting better, more restful sleep, and quicker turnaround times after lifting meant that I was much more effective and productive in my workouts."

—**Kevin,** NASM-CPT, CES, owner of Snodgrass Fitness

Something that may or may not be top of one's mind when it comes to optimal health and performance is **sleep**. No matter the reason might be for your not sleeping well, you'll find that your brain is foggy, or you're a tad bit cranky. You feel sluggish and all you want to do is lay in bed, watch Netflix and snack on sweet stuff or refined carbs all day.

For some people, lack of sleep can become chronic, which can really take a toll on one's quality of life, not to mention lead to chronic diseases. So, are you sleeping well enough to feel and perform your best every day? If the answer is no—which is the case for one in three Americans who are chronically sleep deprived—then continue reading to learn how what you eat can directly affect your sleep habits.

Why Sleep is Important

According to the CDC, adults need 7 or more hours of sleep per night for their best health and wellbeing. Short sleep duration is defined as less than 7 hours of sleep per 24-hour period. Interestingly, if you live in the United States, surveys show that sleep patterns may reflect where you live in the country, with those living in the southeast (GA, SC, AL) and states along the Appalachian Mountains reporting less than 7 hours of sleep a night (more than 40 percent of people living in these states).

The case for adequate sleep is pretty open-and-shut:

- **Sleep plays a vital role in the function of your brain.** Inadequate sleep can disrupt emotions and cognition.

- **Sleep helps regulate your metabolism and appetite.** Lack of restful sleep may increase your risk of becoming overweight due to disrupted hunger and satiety hormones. In fact, poor sleep patterns have been shown to increase overall caloric intake and lead to poor dietary choices.

- **Sleep supports optimal functioning of your immune, hormonal, and cardiovascular systems.** Inflammation can occur without enough sleep, increasing the risk of getting sick, heart issues, and hormonal imbalance.

- **Sleep deprivation has been associated with chronic illness,** including obesity, high blood pressure and Alzheimer's disease.

- **Sleep deprivation can lead to illness,** including training injuries, early fatigue, and suboptimal performance.

- **Sleep helps you live longer.** A 2014 study published in Frontiers in Aging Neuroscience concluded that consistently getting enough sleep is a significant factor in longer life spans.

Plant-Based Diets and Quality Sleep

Plant-based diets are high in complex carbohydrates, including fiber, and isoflavones (more phytonutrients), which may help with quality sleep. Plant-based foods are also sources of **tryptophan** and **melatonin**, which are known to aid in good sleep hygiene. Tryptophan is an amino acid precursor to serotonin (a neurotransmitter) and melatonin (a neurotransmitter-like hormone) production, both of which regulate sleep.

One study found that eating less fiber, more saturated fat and more sugar was associated with lighter, less restorative, and more disrupted sleep in 13 women and 13 men, all normal weight, and an average age of 35 years old. Results show that greater fiber intake predicted more time spent in the stage of deep, slow wave sleep. **In contrast, a higher percentage of energy from saturated fat predicted less slow wave sleep.** Greater sugar intake also was associated with more arousals from sleep. Carbohydrates-rich foods like sweet potatoes, brown rice, and whole grain pasta can stimulate the release of serotonin, which can help you doze off and sleep well throughout the night.

Another study looked at the sleep quality and duration in 106 women, ages 20–75 years, and found that those who ate the most plant-based protein had better sleep quality and significantly longer sleep duration than those who ate animal protein. A Japanese study looked at the isoflavone intake of 1076 women aged 20–78 and found that the higher the isoflavone content the better the sleep quality and longer sleep duration. Plant-based protein sources like soy, beans, and nuts are rich in isoflavones (phytonutrients). These foods are also rich in tryptophan, a precursor to serotonin and melatonin.

A final potential mechanism by which plant-based diets could influence sleep quality is via improvements in body composition. Normal waist circumference, BMI and body fat can reduce the risk of sleep apnea disorders.

Foods high in isoflavones include organic soy, tempeh, edamame, soy milk, miso, lentils, beans, peas, pistachios, peanuts and other nuts. Those containing tryptophan include all of the above, plus sunflower seeds, sesame seeds, pumpkin seeds, sea veggies, leafy greens, walnuts, cauliflower and oat bran. All these foods are also sources of fiber. Plant-based foods high in melatonin include nuts (pistachios being one of the best sources), legumes, tart cherries, pomegranates, tomatoes, mushrooms, peppers, broccoli, oats, barley, strawberries, sunflower seeds, and flax seeds.

Overall, eating a whole food plant-based diet may help with weight management and support serotonin and melatonin production, potentially enhancing sleep quality and duration. If you eat late at night and do not want that meal or snack to interfere with your sleep, choose high fiber, isoflavone-rich, and tryptophan containing foods to help with a good night's sleep like a small bowl of oatmeal with strawberries, a handful of pistachios and cherries, a small kale salad with walnuts and lentils, or unsweetened plant-based yogurt with berries or kiwi.

CHAPTER 19

Supplements

A supplement is exactly that—something which should *supplement* a well-balanced whole food diet, not replace it. A food first attitude is important for optimal health since there are so many components in food that play a part in health (and may even work synergistically, such as how beta carotene and vitamin C enhance the iron absorption in kale). Many supplements are single isolated nutrients or a combination of nutrients that may fill in some gaps and potentially enhance certain aspects of health but are not meant to replace whole foods.

Although supplementation use in athletes has been a topic of concern by health professionals, many experts now take a realistic approach by looking at the risk versus benefit analysis of being safe and effective. Factors like the athletes' age and their sport are also taken into consideration.

Dietary supplements come in many forms, including tablets, capsules, powders, energy bars, and liquids.

They are labeled as dietary supplements and include, among others:

- Vitamin and mineral products
- "Botanical" or herbal products
- Branched chain amino acids and protein supplements
- Enzyme supplements

Supplements have limited regulation, if at all. Federal law does not require dietary supplements to be proven safe to FDA's satisfaction before they are marketed. Once a dietary supplement is on the market, the FDA will monitor any serious adverse events caused by a supplement. It is mandatory that a healthcare professional or the company manufacturing the product report an illness or injury as a result of taking a supplement.

While the FDA requires supplement manufacturers to adhere to Current Good Manufacturing Practices (CGMP or simply GMP), which are intended to ensure the quality and safety of these products, compliance is not always enforced. Therefore, there is no guarantee that the product contains what it claims. The best way to ensure the quality of a product is to look for one that has been third-party tested, which, by the way, is not required by law. However, some supplement manufacturers voluntarily choose to undergo testing to show their commitment to producing high quality products.

One objective indicator of product quality is a Certificate of Analysis (COA), which is given by an independent third-party company, such as NSF (National Sanitation Foundation), USP (United States Pharmacopeia, BSCG (Banned Substances Control Group), or ConsumerLab.

Most products that have been certified by one of these third-party companies have been tested for one or more of the following:

- The supplement contains what is stated on the label and in the amounts listed.

- Products are standardized from batch to batch.

- The supplement is free of harmful levels of contaminants or other potential drug contaminants.

- The product does not contain any undeclared ingredients.

Additionally, if you are a competitive athlete, it can be helpful to look for products that are NSF Certified for Sport. This certification ensures that the product is free of more than 270 substances that are banned or prohibited by most major sports organizations.

The concerns with supplements, even if they have been third-party tested include:

- We may not know their interactions with other supplements.

- They may be toxic with long-term use.

- There could be serious side effects (every individual is different).

- They may not be effective.

- If you are ethically trying to avoid animal products, note that oftentimes supplements are derived from animals or they contain animal byproducts in their "other ingredients" such as gelatin, magnesium stearate or dairy derivatives like casein or caseinate.

Before investing in a supplement, it is important to know what the science says about the supplement's use and in what dose it is potentially effective and safe.

Finally, if you are considering any type of supplementation, know that supplements should be very individualized. Meeting with a registered sports dietitian can help you determine the best supplements and dosing for your performance and body composition goals. Visit eatright.org to find a dietitian that can help with your specific goals.

Branched Chain Amino Acids

There are three types of branched-chain amino acids: leucine, isoleucine, and valine. The unique trait about BCAAs is that they can be metabolized in skeletal muscle, whereas other essential amino acids are metabolized in the liver. Leucine plays an important role in muscle protein synthesis (MPS); that's why it has been proposed that supplementation may play a positive role in muscle protein synthesis and preventing muscle protein breakdown. There is also some research pointing to their role in acting as a fuel for muscles during exercise (although carbohydrates should be your primary fuel and research around BCAAs is inconclusive).

Dosing

Research protocols have used a wide range of dosing strategies however, to get the maximal benefits for muscle protein synthesis and recovery via leucine, a dose of BCAA that provides about 2–3 grams of leucine (this can vary depending on the brand) is suggested.

Side Effects

To date, there have been no adverse side effects reported for BCAAs. One research paper found no toxic effects from daily doses of 1.25 grams per kilogram body weight over twelve months.

Practical Strategies for Supplementation

Enjoy more whole food vegan dietary BCAA sources including lentils, chickpeas, soy, and quinoa. Visit page 42 to get the scoop on foods high in leucine.

B-Alanine

Athletes participating in high intensity sports use a large amount of anaerobic quick energy in the form of ATP (adenosine triphosphate) during intense all-out efforts. There are many reasons why performance can be limited, but one of the major limitations in repeated intensity is the lactate or acid buildup (that lovely burning feeling) in the muscle. One way to buffer that acidosis is through a non-essential amino acid called beta-alanine.

During a short burst of high intensity movement, excess hydrogen ions build up, causing acidosis. One thing that scavenges these hydrogen ions is carnosine, which acts like an antioxidant, preventing fatigue and damage to muscles. Carnosine is what is called a dipeptide, or two amino acids put together. B-alanine and histidine make up carnosine. Only so much carnosine is available during this hydrogen scavenging process. Beta-alanine is used to produce more carnosine. Studies show that 3–6 grams of beta-alanine over four to six weeks may result in 40–60 percent more carnosine. The dose and duration of beta-alanine supplementation seem to be important if you want to make a difference in carnosine content, as well as taking beta-alanine with a meal. Slow-release beta-alanine may also result in greater carnosine synthesis.

Dosing

Research supports taking about 3 to 6 grams of beta-alanine a day (split every 4 hours with a meal) over at least 4 weeks of supplementation, which may increase carnosine stores (30–60 percent) and demonstrate performance benefits. Getting down to specifics, 65 mg per kg of body weight is the ideal dose. For example, a 150-pound person (68 kg) would need 4.4 grams of alanine a day or approximately 1 gram every four hours with meals.

Side Effects

Beta-alanine supplementation currently appears to be safe in healthy populations at recommended doses. However, some people may experience tingling after taking the supplement. Splitting the dose throughout the day and taking smaller doses may help decrease this effect.

Practical Strategies for Supplementation

Beta-alanine has been shown to help with high-intensity training lasting for longer than 60-second bursts or time trials lasting 1–4 minutes. It may be beneficial to athletes who are participating in repetitive high intensity bursts.

Beet Juice

Beets are a source of dietary nitrates that convert to nitric oxide in the body. **Nitric oxide is responsible for dilating blood vessels and delivering more oxygen throughout the body, which may increase the time to exhaustion, improve power output during endurance exercise, regulate muscle contraction, and reduce the cost of energy during exercise.** Plant-based foods that create nitric oxide in the body include beets, garlic, dark chocolate, and leafy greens, to name a few. Beet juice is of particular interest because of its high concentration of nitrates and ease of delivery in a simple beetroot juice shot or through powder.

Dietary nitrate supplementation has been shown to boost performance during high-intensity continuous and intermittent exercise. Research indicates that dietary nitrates may be more effective in sub-elite athletes. It also appears that athletes training or competing at high altitudes (in low oxygen environments) may have particularly good responses to nitrate supplementation. It is unclear if elite athletes might benefit from longer periods, or higher doses, of nitrate supplementation.

Studies have shown mixed results on the effectiveness of beetroot juice and supplements in elite athletes. Elite athletes may benefit from prolonged (more than 3 days) dosing as shown in one study that helped long distance runners. In the small study, elite runners in their 20's were instructed to run to exhaustion on a treadmill, given a red juice supplement for 15 days, and then asked to repeat the treadmill test. Those given beet juice achieved "substantial improvements in the time to exhaustion" compared to those drinking the placebo.

Numerous beetroot supplements are on the market today. However, one study tested various products and found that just 20 percent consistently contained the amount of nitrate required for performance benefit.

Dosing

Research is still needed to determine optimal dosing for specific populations. This lack of consensus and evidence may be due to studies differing in the amount and duration of supplementation, the type of exercise performed, and the training status of the individuals. Doses used in studies vary from approximately 300–600 milligrams of nitrate. Timing of supplementation also varies from a single dose to continuous dose loading.

Athletes using beetroot juice should avoid using mouthwash or gum at the time that they are drinking the juice as they may reduce the bacteria available in the mouth, essential for the conversion of nitrate to nitric oxide.

Side Effects

Those with FODMAPS intolerances may experience mild gut discomfort. Pink colored urine and stool, which is harmless, may also be experienced. Individuals with cardiovascular disease or related risk factors should consult their physician before consuming a high-nitrate diet.

Practical Strategies for Supplementation

The effective nitrate dose studied for performance benefit has been 310–560 milligrams per serving. (There are more than 250 mg of nitrates in 100 grams of beets or beetroot juice.) Beetroot products can be taken 2–3 hours before exercise or daily for up to 14–28 days prior to an event. Current research on whole beets and sports performance benefits is limited. Also, consuming whole beets may be less practical (due to quantity required and gastrointestinal tolerance). Nonetheless, beets are a nutrient-rich food containing phytonutrients, fiber, folate, manganese, vitamin C, and iron. Therefore, I recommend enjoying them daily as part of a plant-based diet. Other nitrate-rich plant-based foods include celery, spinach, arugula, parsley, fennel, leeks, kohlrabi, and collard greens.

If you'd like to try beets or beetroot juice, make sure to trial it during your training phase to assess your gastrointestinal tolerance. If using beet and beetroot juice supplements, choose products that contain an effective dose of nitrates per serving. Consuming more than the recommended amount of nitrate is not recommended.

Tart Cherry Juice

Like beets, cherry juice has also been investigated as a performance enhancer in athletes, also due to cherries' antioxidants and anti-inflammatory compounds. Montmorency, or tart cherries, contains lots of phytonutrients including (fancy names alert!) anthocyanins, flavonoids (quercetin, kaempferol, isorhamnetin), flavanols (catechin, epicatechin), gallic acid equivalents, procyanidins, and phenolic acids. Both tart cherries and sweet cherries contain these compounds; however, tart cherries have higher concentrations.

Tart cherry juice may decrease pain and inflammation and increase recovery after exercise. Studies show that markers of inflammation and oxidative stress are decreased in both strength and endurance athletes, from recreational to well-trained, both male and female, when they drink tart cherry juice daily. Most studies use 8 to 12 ounces of unconcentrated or one ounce of concentrate tart cherry juice twice a day, before and after training or events to promote recovery. For athletes looking to improve recovery and return faster after training or competition, tart cherry may be beneficial.

Tart cherry supplements may also reduce muscle breakdown, muscle soreness and speed up recovery in resistance-trained individuals.

Dosing

What has been used in studies is 8–12 ounces twice a day or one-ounce concentrate twice a day 4–5 days leading up to an event and 2–3 days after the event for optimal recovery in both strength and endurance athletes.

P.S. If you want the fiber, the drink is equivalent to approximately 45 to 60 tart cherries once a day (or 90–120 cherries a day if taken twice a day).

It does also come in powder form. Studies using powdered supplements typically used approximately 480 milligrams per day.

Side Effects

Tart cherry juice is safe for most people; however, it contains high amounts of sorbitol, a type of sugar alcohol that can cause stomach pain and diarrhea for some.

Tart cherry juice also contains quercetin, a plant compound that may interact with certain medications like blood thinners.

Practical Strategies for Supplementation

If you train hard and your focus is getting back into full competition form as fast as possible, then tart cherries may have a beneficial role. It could also be valuable during multi-day events when the ability to recover and perform at a high level is the priority.

Bonus Benefit

Studies also show that tart cherry juice may help with sleep by increasing overall time in bed, total sleep time, and sleep efficiency with the same dose. This may be especially helpful to athletes who have intense training schedules or have to travel for competition, which can cause sleep disturbances. Additionally, unlike melatonin, which may help with sleep quality but not without residual mental and physical fatigue, tart cherry juice may improve cognition and performance.

Caffeine

Caffeine may be the most studied "supplement" on the planet, showing that it is "ergogenic" or "performance-enhancing" in almost every exercise and sporting scenario that has been studied. It is commonly consumed worldwide in a variety of social and sporting settings and was removed from the restricted list of the World Anti-Doping Agency in 2004.

Caffeine stimulates the central nervous system to reduce fatigue and drowsiness. Research has shown that 5–9 milligrams per kg of body weight (340 mg to 613 mg a day for a 150-pound person) can improve endurance and increase muscular strength. The issue with this amount of caffeine is that side effects can occur, such as gastrointestinal upset, nervousness, mental confusion, inability to focus and disturbed sleep.

Good news is on the horizon. More recent research shows that lower caffeine doses, less than 3 milligrams per kilogram of body weight a day can have the same performance effects without the negative side effects. Studies show that lower doses given before exercise, in both men and women, can be beneficial in short and longer endurance events, muscle endurance and strength training, stop-and-go team sports, and individual sports like swimming and golf. It seems that caffeine exerts its effects the most in well-trained athletes who do not include caffeine as part of their regular routine.

Interestingly, studies have also shown that not everyone has the same response to caffeine. You probably know people who can drink coffee before they go to bed and sleep perfectly fine while others cannot have a sip of coffee after 12 noon or else, they will be up all night. It may be in the genes. Liver enzymes are responsible for metabolizing coffee and our genes are responsible for activating the enzyme system to metabolize coffee. Researchers are finding that there are two variants of this gene that activates the enzyme—one variant metabolizes caffeine quickly while the other gene metabolizes caffeine slowly. Which gene do you think you have?

We should give a special nod to green tea, which has approximately 30–50 milligrams of caffeine per 8-ounce cup. It also has phytonutrients (catechin and epigallocatechin–3-gallate or EGCG for short) that act as antioxidants and have been shown to improve cognition, lower the risk of heart disease and diabetes, prevent certain cancers (like breast, prostate, and colon cancer), increase fat metabolism, and alleviate anxiety.

Theanine is an amino acid in green tea that has been shown to boost the neurotransmitters in the brain that make you feel alert yet calm and may help alleviate stress and anxiety. It has also been shown to help with sleep. Studies show that caffeine and theanine may work together to exhibit powerful effects in improving brain function. Due to theanine and the smaller dose of caffeine in green tea compared to coffee, green tea can give you a much milder and different kind of buzz. Many people report having more stable energy and being much more productive when they drink green tea, compared with coffee. (Time green tea appropriately so it does not keep you up at night if you happen to be a slow caffeine metabolizer.)

Dosing

When considering whether to use caffeine as a potential ergogenic aid, athletes may begin with low caffeine doses of ~100–200 milligrams (~1.5–3 mg/kg body weight). Caffeine can be found and rapidly absorbed into the bloodstream through liquids, bars, gels, mouth strips and energy drinks. But why not get all the antioxidant benefits of green tea? Drinking two cups of green tea daily can provide approximately 60–100 milligrams of caffeine.

Side Effects

Side effects can occur with caffeine consumption, such as gastrointestinal upset, nervousness, mental confusion, inability to focus and disturbed sleep. If you are pregnant, limiting caffeine intake to 200 milligrams a day is recommended (there's approximately 73 mg in one 6-ounce cup of coffee).

Practical Strategies for Supplementation

Higher doses do not appear to confer additional advantages. As the response to caffeine consumption is highly variable, athletes need to trial the use of caffeine in training before moving to competition.

Coenzyme Q10 (CoQ10)

You have probably heard about coenzyme Q10—it gets a lot of press for its benefits on prevention of cardiovascular disease. **Another name for coenzyme Q is ubiquinone or ubiquinol (the active form).** It is mostly housed in the mitochondria and is especially abundant in the heart, where it has been shown to help with heart health. It is also associated with improved blood flow and flexibility of the arteries in individuals with heart conditions. Our bodies can make CoQ10, but it decreases as we age. Oxidative stress can also decrease levels (this is where it may benefit athletes). Its main functions are in energy production and protection from free radicals and oxidative cell damage.

In athletes, coenzyme Q10 has been shown to boost athletic performance and decrease inflammation. It is possible that older athletes may benefit the most from supplemental CoQ10 since the enzyme decreases as we age. Research shows that older adults with higher blood levels of CoQ10 tend to be more physically active and have lower levels of oxidative stress, which may help prevent heart disease and cognitive decline. CoQ10 supplements have also been shown to improve muscle strength, vitality, and physical performance in older adults. The amount used in these studies was 100–200 milligrams a day.

Since CoQ10 is involved in the production of energy, it is intriguing to athletes who want to boost performance. CoQ10 supplementation may help to reduce inflammation and expedite recovery.

Dosing

Typically, a 90–200 milligram dose of CoQ10 per day is recommended, though some conditions may require higher doses of 300–600 milligrams. There are two main forms of CoQ10: ubiquinone and ubiquinol. Ubiquinol is often advertised as a better form due to its greater bioavailability. It turns out however, that both seem to be equally effective at raising levels in the body.

Side Effects

Some people who are sensitive to the compound may experience side effects, such as diarrhea, headache, nausea, and skin rashes. It is also recommended to be taken in the morning or afternoon since it may cause insomnia in some folks. Finally, CoQ10 supplements can interact with some common medications, including blood thinners, antidepressants, and chemotherapy drugs.

Practical Strategies for Supplementation

If you are an endurance or strength athlete with an intense training regimen, you could consider taking 100–300 milligrams a day. Dividing the dose (50–150 mg) and taking it twice daily may be most effective.

Creatine

Other than caffeine, creatine might be one of the most well-studied supplements.

Creatine phosphate performs a number of important roles in exercise metabolism, the most well-known being to provide a limited, but quickly accessed, power system to regenerate ATP, the main fuel of the muscle.

Creatine can be obtained from animal sources like meat, poultry and eggs. Our bodies also produce creatine in the kidneys, then it is transported to muscle for use. Muscle creatine levels appear to be lower in vegetarians, indicating that the body's production of creatine may not be sufficient to replace the lack of a dietary source, especially in athletes.

The most basic form of energy in your cells is called adenosine triphosphate or ATP. This is what your body uses for energy, and it runs out pretty quickly during intense exercise. Approximately 95 percent of creatine is stored in the muscles as creatine phosphate, which can replenish ATP during exercise by donating its phosphate, and lead to improved performance, increased strength, and muscle gain.

Hundreds of studies and reviews have been published, with the consensus being that creatine supplementation can increase muscle creatine content and improve exercise capacity and performance. The exercise most likely to benefit from extra creatine is repeated bouts of high-intensity work with short rest periods (e.g., weight training, resistance training, and team and racquet sports). Creatine supplementation may also have a therapeutic role, being able to assist in the gain of muscle mass and strength in elderly and other muscle depleted populations.

Creatine has been shown to increase power in high intensity sports. One study showed 15 grams per day of creatine supplementation for five days to significantly reduce the time needed to complete 40-meter sprints in handball players. Another study found improvements in cycling power after a four-day creatine load with 20 grams a day in males and females. Researchers have also looked at short term versus long term supplementation in swimmers and found that 25 grams of creatine a day for four days improved performance, but continued creatine supplementation of 5 grams per day for two months did not impact performance.

There is consistent evidence that creatine supplementation may improve the recovery between repeated bouts of high-intensity exercise. One study tested explosive power and weightlifting strength and found that 25 grams a day of creatine for one week helped improve explosive jumps and the number of repetitions for bench press. A weight training study found that creatine increased maximum squat and bench press strength.

Creatine loading may be associated with an immediate weight gain of about one kilogram, most likely due to the retention of fluid stored with the creatine inside the cell. Many athletes who continue to gain weight over the next months, often greater than 5 kilograms, claim the weight gain to be mainly muscle. If this is the case, it is likely to be due to the athlete training harder and more effectively during the creatine loading phase.

Endurance exercises are low in intensity and rely less on rapid ATP regeneration. This makes creatine's role less significant. In fact, one study of cross-country runners showed performance impairment following creatine supplementation, which was attributed to the weight gain.

CREATINE STUDIES OF PLANT-BASED EATERS

Are you a vegan strength athlete? One study may be of particular interest to you. Researchers looked at 19 vegetarians (3 vegans) and 30 omnivores and randomly assigned them to either creatine supplementation or a placebo.

As expected, measured creatine levels in the vegetarians were significantly lower compared to the omnivores. After eight weeks on a resistance-training program, all the subjects taking creatine had seen an increase in lean muscle mass and strength compared to placebo. The most significant effect was seen in vegetarians taking creatine who had the highest increase in muscle concentrations of creatine and gained 2.4 kilograms of lean muscle tissue versus 1.9 kilograms of lean muscle tissue for omnivores.

A 2020 systematic review looked at nine studies comparing vegetarians with omnivores taking creatine supplementation and found that vegetarians often had a better response to creatine supplementation with increased creatine in muscles and improved muscle strength and lean tissue.

Brain creatine levels may also be increased with creatine monohydrate supplementation, with several studies having shown improved cognitive processing, which could be valuable for athletes—especially when fatigued.

Dosing

The quickest way to "creatine load" is to take 20–30 g per day for 5–7 days. Typically, these doses are split over the day to sustain plasma creatine levels (for example, 5 grams, four to five times each day). Eating carbohydrates with each dose increases creatine uptake via the stimulatory effects of insulin. Therefore, it is useful to take your creatine doses along with a meal or a carbohydrates-rich snack. Some supplement manufacturers recommend a total daily dose of 3–5 grams a day. This will eventually load the muscle but may take up to 28 days before the muscle is saturated with creatine.

Side Effects

In healthy adults taking recommended doses, clinical trials have not revealed adverse effects. A small number of case studies reporting adverse effects on the kidneys have been published, but these are confounded by pre-existing disease, concomitant medication, other supplement use or extreme unaccustomed exercise. Available data indicate that creatine monohydrate supplementation, when used properly, appears to be safe.

Practical Strategies for Supplementation

Most athletes cycle their creatine supplementation given that the research shows that creatine can be maximized after the loading phase and that individuals with low creatinine levels show the greatest effects with supplementation. However, cycling creatine has not been studied. Based on the research, vegan athletes may see a benefit with 20–30 grams a day of creatine for 5–7 days. There are vegan creatine supplements available. Use your handy know-how to investigate the best supplement for you (look at ingredients, avoid fillers, check for third party testing).

L-Citrulline

L-citrulline increases levels of L-arginine, an amino acid that boosts nitric oxide, dilating blood flow and increasing oxygen delivery to muscles and cells throughout the body. Since the effects of direct arginine supplementation is controversial and arginine supplementation alone has shown limited effects on nitric oxide production, researchers are looking at citrulline as a potential for boosting arginine and nitric oxide production.

Citrulline is a nonessential amino acid (mainly found in watermelon!). The evidence for direct citrulline supplementation is conflicting. Some studies show that it increases nitric oxide production in both strength and endurance athletes while others show no improvement with doses 6–12 grams a day.

Interestingly, arginine has been used in clinical settings to help treat gut injury. Since blood flow is halted to the gut during intense exercise and can cause gastro-intestinal distress and injury, researchers have also been looking at citrulline's role in decreasing intestinal injury in athletes. One study found that 10 grams of citrulline before intense exercise increased blood flow to the gut and decreased intestinal injury.

Dosing

Because evidence is limited, there are no dosing recommendations at this time. As mentioned above, 6–12 grams a day were used in studies with conflicting results.

Side Effects

There have not been any negative side effects reported with the amounts used in the studies.

Strategies for Supplementation

Consuming watermelon before and during training not only naturally provides citrulline, but it also offers lots of water for hydration and electrolytes for electrolyte repletion. For now, eat more watermelon.

Yellow (28 mg citrulline per gram of melon) and orange flesh (14 mg citrulline per gram of melon) melon have more citrulline than red flesh melons (7 mg citrulline per gram of melon). For reference, approximately ⅔ cup is 100 grams so if you eat ⅔ cup of yellow melon you will receive 2.8 grams of citrulline. Very doable!

VEGAN NUTRITION
FOR ATHLETES

CHAPTER 20

Creating a Vegan Athlete Meal Program

"I have been able to switch to a plant-based diet while training for endurance sport while keeping up with breastfeeding (until about 3 months ago) and pregnancy (now). I do love to cook more with plants than I did with meat."

—Meredith, Ultra Runner and endurance athlete

The most common comment I get from folks who want to eat more plant-based for physical performance and health, mental health and overall well-being is: "If you make me vegan meals, I will eat them." It is not that they are opposed to plant-based meals, it is because they either do not know where to start or do not have the time to think about meal prep, let alone prepare it. My goal is to help you get started and make meal planning and preparation as simple as possible. I get it, time is valuable and, unless you are a chef, you do not want to spend all day in the kitchen.

Planning and food preparation, as well as some basic knowledge and kitchen skills, are all helpful when it comes to plant-based eating and these things do require a little bit of time. The good news is that once you carve out a little time to plan and prepare plant-based food you save yourself more time in the long run. Initially, like any change, it may feel out-of-routine and a bit uncomfortable creating new healthy habits around plant-based eating, but I promise you that implementing some simple practices will eventually become part of your lifestyle and get easier with time. You will do them without any thought! Plus, stepping outside of your comfort zone helps you grow and doing something different stimulates the brain. So, consider the new experience an opportunity for growth while you are giving your body needs to optimally perform in your sport and everyday life.

Stock Your Cabinets and Fridge

This plant-based grocery list is meant to be a guide. There are thousands and thousands of edible plants on this planet, so this list is by no means exhaustive. It is just meant to give you an idea of what to stock and includes commonly found foods, at least in the United States. Feel free to adapt the list to make it your own based on what part of the world you live in and what is available in your own backyard (hopefully, you are literally growing food in your own backyard as that's the most nutritious way to enjoy plants!).

Dry foods can have a longer shelf life, therefore, keep them well-stocked in your cabinets. This includes always keeping two to three whole grains, legumes, nuts, and seeds on hand (note that many nuts and seeds should be stored in the refrigerator due to their higher fat content). You can also store nuts, seeds and grains in your freezer and take weekly portions out as needed. Having these items on hand makes meal prep that much easier. Personally, when looking for recipes to make for the week, I like to see what I have on hand and Google away. For example, if I have farro in the cabinet and kale to use in the fridge, I might Google "vegan recipe farro and kale." Then the magical world of Google populates all kinds of goodness. My personal suggestion is to look for recipes that are tried and true, with four to five stars and decent reviews.

You are already eating more plants, which means you are not only making a big impact on your health but also the environment. If you want to further your impact even more, consider purchasing food in bulk whenever possible.

Benefits of buying in bulk:

- **Saves money.** You can save 30 percent to 50 percent by buying natural and organic from the bulk food section.

- **Helps the environment**. Reduce your carbon footprint and minimize what ends up in landfills by using your own reusable bags, containers, or jars.

- **Reduces food waste**. By purchasing only what you need you certainly save money, and you also have less waste. This puts you in control of your purchase quantity and you are not relying on the preset amount packaged by the company.

- **Makes shopping fun**. There are so many varieties of grains, nuts, seeds, flours, dried fruits and more in the bulk food section. Shopping in bulk can be a lot of fun.

- **Allows experimenting with a different food each time you shop in the bulk section**.

- **Allows you to purchase fun reusable bags to fill with bulk foods**. (You can easily find these on Amazon or at your local grocery store.)

- **Helps to stay organized in the kitchen**. Transfer the bulk items to a mason jar when you get home. Do not forget to label the lids with the food item (Been there, done that—I have brought things home and transferred them to a mason jar thinking, "I will remember what that is." Nope, not true. The very next day, I was questioning whether it was wheat berries or kamut or farro that I purchased. Different grains require different amounts of water and cooking time. Do not forget to label.).

On the following pages, you will notice some of the categories we have discussed and the recommended quantities of food you might want to purchase from each category. This will ensure you have plenty of high antioxidant, performance-enhancing, and recovery-promoting foods on hand that you can easily assemble whenever you carve out an hour or two during your week.

Getting the Most Nutrition from Your Food

A few questions often arise when it comes to purchasing and cooking food: Are frozen fruits okay to purchase? Do I need to start with dried beans or is canned okay? What's the best way to cook vegetables so they retain their nutrition or is it better to eat them raw?

Choose Two to Three Whole Grains

Amaranth	Farro	Quinoa
Brown Rice	Kamut	Red Rice
Bulgur Wheat	Millet	Wheat Berries
Barley	Oats	

Choose At Least Two Types of Legumes

Adzuki Beans	Fava Beans	Mung Beans
Black Beans	Green Peas	Navy Beans
Black Eyed Peas	Kidney Beans	Pinto Beans
Chickpeas	Lentils	

Choose One or Two Starchy Vegetables

Acorn Squash	Purple Potato	Yam
Butternut Squash	Red Potato	
Pumpkin	Sweet Potato	

Choose Two to Three Aromatics

Garlic	Onion
Ginger	Shallots

Choose Two to Three "Other" Veggies

Asparagus	Cucumber	Red Pepper
Beets	Fennel	Squash
Carrots	Mushrooms	Tomatoes
Celery	Okra	

Choose Two Leafy Greens

Mizuno	Red Leaf Lettuce	Spinach
Radicchio	Romaine	

Choose Two to Three Cruciferous Veggies

Arugula	Cauliflower	Radish
Bok Choy	Collard Greens	Red Cabbage
Broccoli	Kale	Watercress
Brussel Sprouts	Mustard Greens	

Choose Two to Three Seeds

Chia	Hemp Seed	Sesame Seeds
Flaxseeds	Pumpkin Seeds	Sunflower Seeds

Choose Two to Three Nuts

Almonds	Peanuts (technically	Pine Nuts
Brazil Nuts	a legume)	Pistachios
Cashews	Pecans	Walnuts

Choose One or Two Berries

Blackberries	Cranberries	Strawberries
Blueberries	Currants	
Boysenberries	Raspberries	

Choose Two or Three Other Fruits

Apples	Kiwi	Plum
Bananas	Mango	Pomegranates
Dates	Oranges	Prunes
Figs	Peach	Watermelon
Grapefruit	Pears	
Guava	Pineapple	

Optional Items (Recommended for Variety and Nutrition)
Choose One or Two Soy Foods

Edamame	Tempeh
Miso	Tofu

Choose One or Two Sea Vegetables

Dulse	Kelp Seasoning	Wakame
Dulse Flakes	Nori	
Kelp	Spirulina	

Personal Recommendations and Must-Haves

Avocado
Dark Chocolate (70 percent or higher, organic, Fair Trade)

Choose At Least Two Herbs

Basil	Lemon Grass	Rosemary
Chives	Mint	Thyme
Cilantro	Oregano	
Dill	Parsley	

First, frozen fruits and vegetables can sometimes be more nutritious than fresh because they're harvested and frozen immediately when they're ripe, which preserves nutrition. Harvesting when they're ripe also means they'll most likely have more flavor. Compare this to fruit and veggies that are harvested before they ripen because they need to sit on transportation for days, or perhaps weeks, before they make it to the grocery store shelves where there's more time to sit before you purchase them. This process can rob produce of their flavor and nutrition. This is one reason why it's also good to purchase in-season and local or regional produce. It's not only more nutritious, but it's also often tastier and better for the planet since the food doesn't have to travel as far.

Regarding canned products, they're a quick and easy way to access many foods that you may not have time to prepare. Soaking beans overnight, followed by draining then cooking them doesn't require a lot of preparation time (I typically let them cook them while I'm doing things around the house or in a Zoom meeting), but it does require a little planning. For example, if you want to have bean tacos for dinner, you'll need to plan ahead a bit to soak and cook the beans. When you prepare something in a pinch, canned products can be helpful. Just choose BPA-free to avoid the harmful plastic chemicals that can leach into the cans.

With regard to cooked versus raw or steamed versus boiled, it can depend on the plant and nutrients. Water soluble nutrients like vitamin C are often lost in cooking whereas fat soluble nutrients are often enhanced through cooking. For example, the carotenoids in carrots and tomatoes are more bioavailable when they're cooked while the vitamin C in leafy greens is preserved when they're consumed raw. Personally, I don't digest cruciferous vegetables, like broccoli and cauliflower, well if I eat them raw. However, I enjoy them immensely and digest them fine if they're lightly steamed or sautéed.

Bottom line is to eat your veggies the way you like them, whether they're cooked or raw, steamed or roasted. (Sorry, this doesn't mean going to town on French fries and other fried veggies.) Experiment with a variety of ways to eat veggies before you say no. For example, you also may not enjoy raw broccoli, but that's not to say you won't love it in vegan mac and cheese or enjoy puréed creamy broccoli soup. Try a variety of cooking methods or different cuts before you say no to that veggie.

Getting Started

As an athlete with specific performance goals, every bite counts. **The first step to eating a well-balanced plant-based diet is to have plant-based staples on hand so that you can easily prepare a meal or snack on-the-fly or pre-plan by batch making meals for the week.**

Some examples of nutritious meals and snacks you can prepare quickly include smoothies and smoothie bowls, grain bowls, nut or seed butter and fruit spread sandwiches, plant-based yogurt and fruit, or hummus and whole-grain crackers.

Grain Bowls

One way to create a foundation that will fuel, replenish, and energize you every single day is to create grain bowls. To make grain-bowl prep super-duper easy, you might consider batch cooking one day a week. I know this sounds like a full day of kitchen prep, but trust me, it will only require one hour out of your week, and you can often do this while you are busy doing other things around the house or working in front of your computer.

Batch Cooking Grains

Batch cooking is extremely helpful and a huge time-saver in the kitchen. Select one day out of the week when you can prepare one large batch of grains that can be stored away in the refrigerator or in individual containers in the freezer, so you have grains all week or month long. For me, batch cooking happens when I wake up in the morning. There is an hour when I am enjoying my morning tea or coffee while answering emails. Before I hop on the computer I boil water, add grains, and cover while simmering until they are done. If you have an Instant Pot, hooray! You have just cut your cook time down significantly.

When the grains are finished, not only do I have ⅓ of my meal for the day and days ahead prepared, but I also silently give myself a high-five because I have not even fully started the day and a significant part of meal prep is complete (those of you who love to check things off your list, you get me here, right?). Whole grains can include brown or black rice, farro, buckwheat, wheat berries, kamut, millet, amaranth, or quinoa. You could also substitute starchy vegetables for the grains as your carbohydrate of choice like purple or red potatoes, sweet potatoes, or yucca.

Protein for Your Grain Bowl

Next is your protein (although, many grains are jam-packed with protein and could essentially count as your protein). While you are cooking your grains, you could also cook your beans (or simply open the can and drain). If you had good intentions on soaking your beans but completely forgot then those back-up canned beans will work perfectly for your grain bowl. Stock up on BPA-free canned beans from the grocery store. With cans of black beans, chickpeas, pinto beans, lentils, and great northern beans in your pantry, the most time-consuming part of making this meal will be operating the can opener.

You could also consider lentils or split peas, which require no soaking, just boiling and take only about 30 minutes to cook. If you really want to save time, add 1 cup of lentils and 1 cup of quinoa to the same pot with 3 cups of water or veggie broth (for more flavor), bring to a boil then simmer, covered, for 30 minutes and you have both your grain and protein ready to go. Beans, peas, and lentils can all be used as your protein. Other foods that will provide lots of protein include tofu, tempeh, nuts, and seeds.

What about plant-based meats? **Plant-based meats are a greener alternative to traditional meat.** They are a simple solution to replacing meat on consumer's plates because they require little preparation and offer flavors, textures, and protein similar to that of traditional meat. Are plant-based meats of the same nutritional value as quinoa black bean burgers made with vegetables and whole food ingredients? No, they are not, but they are a step in the right direction for the planet and for health. To offset their often high sodium content, minimize added salt or sodium in other foods or meals.

Veggies for Your Grain Bowl

Next, you want to add your colorful veggies. **Grains and beans provide phytonutrients that will decrease inflammation and expedite recovery; however, vegetables will provide even more, as well as a diverse range of nutrients.** Add some pre-washed greens to your grain bowl, red onion, carrots, bell pepper, radish, beets—the options are pretty endless! I would suggest adding three plant-based colors or veggies to each grain bowl (and to any meal) to ensure that you are getting a variety of fiber and phytonutrients for optimal health. If frozen veggies are your jam, then hooray! Frozen veggies (and fruits) often have even more nutrition because they are frozen immediately after harvest, meaning they retain their nutritional value. Oftentimes, frozen vegetables can be a cost-saver as well.

Dressings and Sauces

Having dressings and sauces on hand is another bonus, especially when you are running low on time. Most dressings and sauces take only minutes to prepare. If you have that hour set aside to prepare your grains, then you could use that hour to make one or two dressings or sauces while the grains are cooking. **A sauce or dressing will elevate any grain bowl and transform it from bland to super tasty in a matter of seconds.** Having two or three dressings or sauces on hand is good for those of you who like variety throughout the week. See Page 203 for sauce and dressing recipes.

Finishing Touches

Finishing touches on grain bowls can also transform them into even more deliciousness plus more nutrition. Add nuts and seeds like slivered almonds, cashews, or pistachios. Or add seeds like pumpkin, sunflower, hemp, or sesame seeds. Adding herbs not only provides flavor but do not forget that those herbs are plants too, meaning they are packed with vitamins, minerals, and phytonutrients that fight inflammation, support performance, and expedite recovery, among other things. Add fresh cilantro, basil, chives or parsley or dried herbs like oregano, rosemary, or thyme.

Below are a few grain bowl suggestions to get you started:

- Wheat berries, chickpeas, kale, purple onion, and radish, sunflower seeds

- Whole wheat pasta, edamame, spinach, tomatoes, mushrooms, pine nuts

- Brown rice, black beans, asparagus, cauliflower, carrots, pumpkin seeds

- Quinoa, tofu, broccoli, red bell pepper, bok choy, cashews

Think in Threes

Making changes to your life, whether it is diet, a move, marriage, kids or anything else, can be stressful. When thinking about the complete overhaul it can seem overwhelming and daunting, to say the least. I remember when I was starting a chocolate company. I created a URL for the website, which was exciting. But taking the chocolates I was creating in my kitchen to a sellable product with packaging, getting it into stores, creating a website and more was paralyzing. Figuring out the packaging alone was paralyzing.

Instead of focusing on the end result and scattering my mind with all of the details in between, I had to think about what was small and attainable. What can I do today that can make a difference and get me closer to that end goal? I started making lists of 3's, which felt doable to me. It was something as simple as calling a graphic designer to get a packaging quote to writing a description of the chocolate on my website to having a friend taste the chocolate for feedback.

All three of those things are practical and easy to check off my to-do list for the day. Each day I had a list of threes, and by the end of each week I accomplished a lot that would get me closer to launching a chocolate company. Eventually, what once seemed daunting seemed completely attainable and simple-to-do once the goals were broken down into easy steps. I use this formula for everything in life now (even writing this book!). Little steps add up quickly and can lead to big results.

Here are my suggested lists of 3's for you as you're either making changes, trying to eat more plant-based foods or if you want to optimize your already plant-based diet. But feel free to create your own list of 3's that works best for you!

Create three small goals a week. If you are thinking of eating more plants or going vegan for your health or the planet, here are some small steps you can take today that will lead to big long term positive changes:

- Swap a bean burger for a regular burger one day a week.
- Swap veggie broth for meat broth or flax eggs for regular eggs.
- Try Meatless Mondays.
- Eat one plant-based meal a day.
- Experiment with one plant-based recipe a week.
- Add leafy greens to meals (add greens to a sandwich, smoothie, or pasta).

Shoot for three colors per meal. In the case of beans, whole grains, and mushrooms, browns, and tans count. Choose reds (tomato, strawberries, peppers, radish), purples (beets, red onion, cabbage, potato, grapes), greens (arugula, broccoli, spinach, kale, kiwi, avocado, apple), oranges (pepper, citrus, sweet potato, squash), and yellows (banana, lemon, pineapple, squash). For example, start your morning with color by making avocado toast (green) with spinach (more green) tomato (red) and purple onion. Or blend a smoothie with banana (yellow), berries (red and purple), kale (green), and chia. Or make oatmeal with flax (tan), berries (red and purple) and a teaspoon of matcha or Moringa powder (green!).

Choose three recipes to make. Doing this over the course of a month may be more doable, but strive to find your favorite recipe blogs or invest in one or two cookbooks (see page 223 for suggestions) and choose three recipes to try this week or throughout the month. Balance out simple, less than 30-minute recipes with recipes that take a little more time. Or keep them all simple! There are no rules here. Choose recipes that look appealing and doable for you. One time-saving tip is to choose recipes that have similar ingredients so that if two recipes call for quinoa, you can double the batch of quinoa you are making so you are only making it once for two meals. It is also helpful to choose recipes with similar ingredients when grocery shopping. Choose three recipes for the week or the month, make a shopping list based on what you already have on hand and what you need, shop, and prepare whatever you can ahead of time so that the actual meal prep is efficient and takes less time.

Swap three proteins one week. If you do not want to make a single change to your meals but just want to swap meat and dairy out with plant-based foods then consider swapping three meat or dairy-based meals out with plant-based protein. For example, substitute a bean burger in place of a regular burger. Or grab yourself some plant-based "chicken" (my personal favor is No Evil Foods) to eat in place of regular chicken. Enjoy tempeh, a "meaty" substitute for the meat on your plate. Swap plant-based milk for dairy milk.

Make three sauces or dressings for the week. Trust me, you will thank yourself, especially if you are a sauce and dressing lover, if you have two to three sauces or dressings ready to go for the week. Having a homemade sauce or dressing ready to go makes meal prep simple and adding them to meals makes the dish extra yummy! (See page 175 for recipes!)

Sample Meal Plans

Everyone is an individual, and no one meal plan fits all. **That's why the meal plans below are meant to be guides to give you screenshots of plant-based eating.** If you are a strength athlete and feel you need more protein, feel free to add protein powder to your regiment or incorporate plant-based meat made with vital wheat gluten or pea protein once or twice a week. Since these foods are processed, I would not suggest them for every meal, but they can certainly fit into a healthy meal plan since they can provide a dedicated source of protein.

If you are an endurance athlete you might want to alter the carbohydrates and fat ratios so that you are receiving a higher percentage of carbohydrates, especially during and after training when glucose needs are high and glycogen repletion is a priority. If you have a nut allergy, consider substituting sunflower or pumpkin seeds for nuts. If you tend to eat a mid-morning snack and not an afternoon snack, then swap the snack times I have listed. If you like to enjoy smaller meals 5–6 times a day, then split your lunch or dinner in half. Finally, if you choose to follow the meal guides below, customize the quantity and timing of meals to meet your specific training and performance regimen and goals.

Suggested alterations for endurance athletes needing a higher percentage of carbohydrates: Increase your portions of carbohydrates-rich foods like fruit, sweet potatoes, oatmeal, quinoa, rice, and other whole grains.

Suggested alterations for strength training athletes needed more protein: Boost protein intake by using plant-based meat (often an isolated source of protein) and using quality (third-party tested) protein powders.

Suggested alterations for those sticking to a lower fat diet: Plant-based proteins like avocado, nuts, seeds, tofu and tempeh can contribute to a significant amount of fat. While the type of fat found in plant products is healthier than the type found in animal products, fat, in general, can contribute to significant calories. Therefore, if you're managing weight for health reasons, consider decreasing the portion sizes of those high fat foods, like avocado, nuts, seeds, tofu, and tempeh.

1800-Calorie Meal Plan

Breakfast

1 cup oatmeal, 1 cup soy milk, ½ cup blueberries, 1 tablespoon flax meal, 1 ounce almonds

- 522 calories, 62 grams carbohydrates (47 grams net carbohydrates), 15 grams fiber, 22 grams protein, 23 grams fat

Lunch

Salad Bowl, made from 2 cups leafy greens, ½ cup cooked quinoa, ½ cup cooked lentils, 2 radishes (sliced), ¼ cup beets, 1 tablespoon sunflower seeds, 2 tablespoons Green Goddess dressing (page 204)

- 418 calories, 52.5 grams carbohydrates (39.5 grams net carbohydrates), 13 grams fiber, 17.5 grams protein, 17 grams fat

Snack

1 apple, 1 tablespoon peanut butter

- 189 calories, 27 grams carbohydrates (21 grams net carbohydrates), 6 grams fiber, 4 grams protein, 8 grams fat

Dinner

Stir Fry, made from 1 cup cooked brown rice, 3 ounces firm tofu, 1 cup broccoli, 1 cup red pepper, 2 tablespoons teriyaki sauce

- 465 calories, 83 grams carbohydrates (70 grams net carbohydrates), 13 grams fiber, 22 grams protein, 8 grams fat

Snack

6 ounces plant-based yogurt, 1 cup berries

- 200 calories, 43 grams carbohydrates (38 grams net carbohydrates), 5 grams fiber, 2 grams protein, 4 grams fat

---

TOTAL: 1794 calories, 267.5 grams carbohydrates (215.5 grams net carbohydrates), 52 grams fiber, 67.5 grams protein, 52 grams fat

2000-Calorie Meal Plan

Breakfast

Smoothie made from 1 banana, 1 cup berries, 1 handful kale, 1 tablespoon almond butter, 1 cup soy milk, 2 tablespoons hemp seeds

- 422 calories, 57 grams carbohydrates (45 grams net carbohydrates), 12 grams fiber, 19 grams protein, 18 grams fat

Lunch

Chickpea Salad Wrap with 1 cup chickpea salad, 1 whole grain tortilla, leafy greens, red onion, tomato

- 407 calories, 63 grams carbohydrates (48 grams net carbohydrates), 15 grams fiber, 19 grams protein, 15 grams fat

Snack

8 ounces Kite Hill protein plant-based yogurt, 1 cup chopped fruit, 2 tablespoons homemade granola

- 333 calories, 44 grams carbohydrates (51 grams net carbohydrates), 5 grams fiber, 18 grams protein, 12 grams fat

Dinner

1 serving Champion Chili (page 193) plus 2 tablespoons nutritional yeast

- 404 calories, 56 grams carbohydrates (37 grams net carbohydrates), 19 grams fiber, 31.5 grams protein, 8 grams fat

Snack

Endurance Banana Bread (page 209), 1 cup cherries

- 432 calories, 76 grams carbohydrates (62 grams net carbohydrates), 10 grams fiber, 10 grams protein, 12.5 grams fat

TOTAL: 1998 calories, 296 grams carbohydrates (243 grams net carbohydrates), 61 grams fiber, 95.5 grams protein, 65.5 grams fat

2200-Calorie Meal Plan

Breakfast

3 Go for the Gold Pancakes (page 179), 2 tablespoons strawberry jam, 2 tablespoons cashew butter, 1 tablespoon maple syrup

- 496 calories, 50 grams carbohydrates (43 grams net carbohydrates), 7 grams fiber, 18 grams protein, 16 grams fat

Lunch

Hummus wrap with ½ cup hummus, 3 ounces grilled tempeh, carrots, leafy greens, cucumber and whole grain tortilla, 1 apple

- 628 calories, 85 grams carbohydrates (68 grams net carbohydrates), 15 grams fiber, 29.5 grams protein, 23 grams fat

Snack

10 whole grain crackers, 2 ounces bean spread, microgreens, 1 orange

- 265 calories, 41 grams carbohydrates (33 grams net carbohydrates), 8 grams fiber, 8 grams protein, 9 grams fat

Dinner

Chickpea pasta (4 ounces) with 1 cup red sauce and 1 cup broccoli

- 565 calories, 94 grams carbohydrates (69 grams net carbohydrates), 26 grams fiber, 35 grams protein, 12 grams fat

Snack

Strawberry Milkshake made from 1 cup soy milk blended with 1 cup strawberries, 1 banana, 2 tablespoons flax meal

- 289 calories, 47 grams carbohydrates (34 grams net carbohydrates), 13 grams fiber, 13 grams protein, 8 grams fat

TOTAL: 2243 calories, 317 grams carbohydrates (247 grams net carbohydrates), 69 grams fiber, 103.5 grams protein, 68 grams fat

2400-Calorie Meal Plan

Breakfast

Avocado toast made from 2 slices whole grain bread, 1 avocado (smashed), sliced tomato, arugula, 1 tablespoon hemp seeds, 1 tablespoon kimchi, 1 cup mango

- 538 calories, 92 grams carbohydrates (68 grams net carbohydrates), 24 grams fiber, 13 grams protein, 19 grams fat

Lunch

Grain bowl made from 1 cup cooked lentils, 1 cup cooked amaranth, 2 cups mixed veggies, 2 tablespoons Green Goddess Dressing (page 204)

- 707 calories, 116.5 grams carbohydrates (94 grams net carbohydrates), 22.5 grams fiber, 39 grams protein, 16 grams fat

Snack

1 banana, 2 tablespoons peanut butter

- 292 calories, 34 grams carbohydrates (28 grams net carbohydrates), 6 grams fiber, 9 grams protein, 16 grams fat

Dinner

1 serving Ironman Mac N Cheese (page 190), side salad with red leaf lettuce, tomato, red onion, 1 cup cubed sweet potato, and radish, light drizzle olive oil and lemon juice

- 685 calories, 93 grams carbohydrates (75 grams net carbohydrates), 18 grams fiber, 33 grams protein, 24 grams fat

Snack

1 Brazil nut, 1 cup mixed berries, 6 ounces Kite Hill protein plant-based yogurt

- 210 calories, 19 grams carbohydrates (31 grams net carbohydrates), 4.5 grams fiber, 14 grams protein, 10 grams fat

---

TOTAL: 2432 calories, 354.5 grams carbohydrates (296 grams net carbohydrates), 75 grams fiber, 108 grams protein, 85 grams fat

2600-Calorie Meal Plans

Breakfast

Breakfast burrito made from 1 large whole grain tortilla, ½ cup black beans, ¼ cup salsa, 1 cup spinach, ½ avocado
- 570 calories, 89 grams carbohydrates (66 grams net carbohydrates), 23 grams fiber, 21 grams protein, 18 grams fat

Lunch

Tempeh "BLT" made from 2 slices whole grain bread, 4 ounces tempeh bacon, leafy greens, tomato, 2 tablespoons vegan mayo
- 578 calories, 55 grams carbohydrates (44 grams net carbohydrates), 11 grams fiber, 33 grams protein, 17 grams fat

Snack

No-Bake Nutty Seedy Bars (page 210)
- 436 calories, 44 grams carbohydrates (35 grams net carbohydrates), 9 grams fiber, 24 grams protein, 21 grams fat

Dinner

Grilled Tofu Skewers made with 6 ounces tofu, 1 cup mushrooms, 1 cup red peppers, ½ cup onion, 1 cup pineapple, 1 cup black rice, 2 tablespoons tamari marinade
- 629 calories, 104 grams carbohydrates (88 grams net carbohydrates), 16 grams fiber, 33 grams protein, 13 grams fat

Snack

1 serving Cool Down Chia Pudding (page 213), 1 cup berries
- 406 calories, 55 grams carbohydrates (41 grams net carbohydrates), 14 grams fiber, 13 grams protein, 16 grams fat

TOTAL: 2619 calories, 347 grams carbohydrates (274 grams net carbohydrates), 73 grams fiber, 124 grams protein, 85 grams fat

2800-Calorie Meal Plans

Breakfast

Recovery Smoothie (page 183), ½ cup oatmeal, ½ cup plant milk, 1 scoop of plant-based protein powder

- 586 calories, 80 grams carbohydrates (56 grams net carbohydrates), 18 grams fiber, 40 grams protein, 18 grams fat

Lunch

Salad Bowl made with 2 cups leafy greens, 1 cup cooked quinoa, 1 cup edamame, 1 cup broccoli, sliced radish, 1 tablespoon pumpkin seeds, orange slices, Ultra Lemon Dijon Dressing (page 206)

- 727 calories, 108 grams carbohydrates (77 grams net carbohydrates), 32.5 grams fiber, 39 grams protein, 19 grams fat

Snack

½ cup homemade trail mix with nuts and dried fruit, 1 cup plant-based yogurt

- 567 calories, 81 grams carbohydrates (71 grams net carbohydrates), 10 grams fiber, 12 grams protein, 26 grams fat

Dinner

Cross Country Lentil Burgers (page 196), whole grain bun, lettuce, tomato, vegan mayo

- 575 calories, 92 grams carbohydrates (68 grams net carbohydrates), 24 grams fiber, 21 grams protein, 18 grams fat

Snack

1 cup oatmeal, ¾ cup soy milk, 1 cup berries

- 411 calories, 69 grams carbohydrates (56 grams net carbohydrates), 13 grams fiber, 18 grams protein, 8 grams fat

TOTAL: 2866 calories, 430 grams carbohydrates (328 grams net carbohydrates), 97.5 grams fiber, 130 grams protein, 89 grams fat

3000-Calorie Meal Plans

Breakfast

Overnight oats made from 1 cup oatmeal, 1½ cups plant milk, 2 tablespoons pecans, 1 sliced banana, 1 tablespoon maple syrup, 1 teaspoon cinnamon

- 677 calories, 97 grams carbohydrates (84 grams net carbohydrates), 13 grams fiber, 25 grams protein, 22 grams fat

Snack

Whole grain tortilla, ½ cup refried black beans, salsa, Romaine leaves

- 233 calories, 43 grams carbohydrates (35 grams net carbohydrates), 9 grams fiber, 9 grams protein, 3 grams fat

Lunch

Stamina Beet Burgers (page 195) using 1 whole grain bun, vegan mayo, leafy greens, tomato, onion, ½ avocado

- 636 calories, 58 grams carbohydrates (42 grams net carbohydrates), 16 grams fiber, 25 grams protein, 25 grams fat

Snack

Baked sweet potato, 1 cup lentils, tahini and lemon sauce

- 488 calories, 83 grams carbohydrates (64 grams net carbohydrates), 19 grams fiber, 24 grams protein, 9 grams fat

Dinner

Long, Slow and Steady Tempeh Farro Bowl (page 201)

- 635 calories, 76 grams carbohydrates (58 grams net carbohydrates), 18 grams fiber, 44 grams protein, 22 grams fat

Snack

1 cup baked crunchy chickpeas, 1 cup kale with drizzle olive oil and lemon juice, chopped apples

- 346 calories, 59 grams carbohydrates (44 grams net carbohydrates), 14 grams fiber, 11 grams protein, 9 grams fat

TOTAL: 3015 calories, 416 grams carbohydrates (327 grams net carbohydrates), 89 grams fiber, 138 grams protein, 90 grams fat

THE
RECIPES

Morning Fuel

Easy grab 'n go breakfasts might be quick stovetop oatmeal or peanut butter and jelly on toast or maybe yogurt and granola. These are all fantastic, however, I wanted to share some of my personal favorite breakfast recipes for when I have a bit more time. Although the Nut Runner's Fuel and Go For the Gold Pancakes actually take very little time. Plus, there are some recipes you can prepare ahead of time like the Adventure Athlete's Morning Oatmeal. Have fun getting energized with these nutrient-powered breakfasts that could also easily sub for post-training meals!

THE ADVENTURE ATHLETE'S MORNING OATMEAL

SERVES: **6** · PREP TIME: **10 MINUTES** · COOKING TIME: **25 MINUTES**

FLAX MEAL EGG

2 tablespoons flax meal

6 tablespoons water

WET INGREDIENTS

1 cup plant-based milk, unsweetened

2 tablespoons apple cider vinegar

½ cup ripe banana, mashed

¼ cup maple syrup

2 teaspoons vanilla extract

DRY INGREDIENTS

2 cups organic rolled oats

¼ cup almond meal

2 teaspoons baking powder

2 teaspoons ground cinnamon

¼ teaspoon ground ginger

¼ teaspoon ground nutmeg

2 pinches salt

1 cup chopped pears

¾ cup chopped pecans

1. Preheat the oven to 350°F and line muffin tins with paper liners or spray with oil.

2. Make the flax meal egg: Add the flax meal and water to a small bowl, stir, and set aside to gel.

3. Mix together the wet ingredients: In a medium bowl mix together the milk, apple cider vinegar, banana, maple syrup, and vanilla extract.

4. Mix together the dry ingredients: In a large bowl, mix together the rolled oats, almond meal, baking powder, cinnamon, ginger, nutmeg, and salt.

5. Combine the wet ingredients with the dry ingredients.

6. Fold in the flax meal egg.

7. Stir in the pears and pecans.

8. Pour the batter into the muffin tins, filling ¾ full and bake for 25 minutes.

9. Remove from the oven and allow to cool for 5 minutes before serving. Store leftovers in the refrigerator for up to 5 days.

Per serving: 313 calories, 7 grams protein, 41 grams total carbohydrates (33 grams net carbohydrates), 15.5 grams fat, 7 grams fiber, 34 milligrams sodium

.5 mcg B12, 132 mg calcium, 2.5 mg iron, 90 mg magnesium

7 mcg selenium, 1.8 mg zinc

NUT RUNNER'S FUEL

SERVES: 4 · PREP TIME: **10 MINUTES** · COOKING TIME: **12 MINUTES**

GRANOLA

½ cup chopped raw almonds
½ cup chopped raw walnuts
½ cup chopped raw pecans
¼ cup pumpkin seeds
¾ teaspoon cinnamon
1 cup organic rolled oats
1 tablespoon coconut oil
¼ cup maple syrup
1 teaspoon vanilla extract
⅛ teaspoon salt

FRUIT AND MILK

1–2 cups fruit of choice
   (berries, sliced banana,
   apples, cherries)
plant-based milk,
   unsweetened

1. Preheat oven to 350°F and line a baking sheet with parchment paper.

2. Place the almonds, walnuts, pecans, pumpkin seeds, and cinnamon in a large bowl.

3. Grind the oats into a coarse meal in a food processor or grinder.

4. Add the oats to the bowl with the nuts and stir to combine.

5. Melt the coconut oil then, in a small bowl, mix together the coconut oil, maple syrup and vanilla extract.

6. Pour the mixture over the oats, nuts, and pumpkin seed mixture.

7. Mix well until the nuts, oats, and seeds are coated.

8. Spread out evenly on the baking sheet and lightly sprinkle with salt.

9. Bake for 12 minutes, stirring halfway through. Let cool for 10 minutes before serving.

10. Divide the granola between two bowls. Divide the fruit between the bowls and pour the desired amount of milk over top. Store leftover granola in a container on the countertop for up to 7 days or in the refrigerator for up to 2 weeks.

Per serving: 507 calories, 15 grams protein, 44 grams total carbohydrates (34.5 grams net carbohydrates), 34 grams fat, 9.5 grams fiber, 121 milligrams sodium

1.5 mcg B12, 252 mg calcium, 13.25 mg iron, 177 mg magnesium, 9 mcg selenium, 3.2 mg zinc

GO FOR THE GOLD PANCAKES

SERVES: **4** · PREP TIME: **5 MINUTES** · COOKING TIME: **10 MINUTES**

CHIA EGG
2 tablespoons chia seeds
6 tablespoons water

WET INGREDIENTS
1 cup plant-based milk,
   unsweetened
2 tablespoons apple cider
   vinegar
1 teaspoon vanilla extract
¼ cup ripe banana, mashed

DRY INGREDIENTS
1 ½ cups buckwheat flour
¼ cup coconut sugar
2 teaspoons baking powder
1 teaspoon ground cinnamon
¼ teaspoon salt

FRUIT
¾ cup blueberries

1. Make the chia egg: Add the chia seeds and water to a small bowl. Stir and set aside to gel.

2. Add the milk, apple cider vinegar, vanilla extract, and banana to a medium bowl and mix until combined.

3. Add all of the dry ingredients to a large bowl and mix to combine.

4. Transfer the wet ingredients to the dry ingredients and stir, but don't overmix.

5. Fold in the chia egg and blueberries.

6. Make the pancakes: Spray a stovetop pan or griddle with oil to prevent the pancakes from sticking. Heat the pan on medium heat. With a ladle, pour four 4" pancakes onto the griddle. Cook on each side for about 1–2 minutes until golden brown on the bottom then flip to cook the other side until golden brown.

7. Transfer the cooked pancakes to a dish then continue the same process with the remaining batter. This should make approximately 12 pancakes.

8. Top with your favorite nut butter and fruit. Store leftovers in the refrigerator for up to 5 days. Reheat on the stovetop.

Per serving: 256 calories, 8.5 grams protein, 51 grams total carbohydrates (43.5 grams net carbohydrates), 4 grams fat, 7.5 grams fiber, 418 milligrams sodium

0.75 mcg B12, 536 mg calcium, 3.25 mg iron, 148 mg magnesium, 7 mcg selenium, 1.8 mg zinc

WARRIOR BREAKFAST BOWL

2 cups cooked quinoa

1 cup shredded carrots

1 medium tomato, diced

2 cups chopped spinach

1 large avocado, cubed

½ cup diced red onion

¼ cup diced olives

¼ cup hummus (plain or your favorite flavor)

2 teaspoons olive oil

1 large lemon, juiced

2 tablespoons chopped parsley

Salt to taste

Black pepper, to taste

1. In a large bowl, add quinoa, carrots, tomato, spinach, avocado, onion and olives. Mix well.

2. In a small bowl, add hummus, oil, and lemon. Mix well. Add 1–2 tablespoons of water if you would like a thinner consistency to pour over the salad.

3. Drizzle hummus and lemon over salad and mix well. Sprinkle with parsley, salt and pepper if desired.

4. Dish into two bowls and enjoy! Store leftovers in the refrigerator for up to 5 days.

Per serving: 578 calories, 16.5 grams protein, 74.5 grams total carbohydrates (57 grams net carbohydrates), 26.5 grams fat, 17.5 grams fiber, 497 milligrams sodium

0.0 mcg B12, 171 mg calcium, 6.7 mg iron, 186 mg magnesium, 10.5 mcg selenium, 3.5 mg zinc

SMOOTHIES AND SMOOTHIE BOWLS

Smoothies and smoothie bowls might be the simplest and most fun way to pack in the most nutrients in the smallest amount of space when you're running low on time. You can disguise greens if you don't incorporate enough, boost protein if you are looking to gain muscle, or sneak in adaptogens through powders and tinctures. Plus, if you are an artistic smoothie bowl maker (I am not) then you have social media worthy photos that are pure eye candy!

POWER PACKED SMOOTHIE BOWL

SERVES: **2** • PREP TIME: **5 MINUTES** • COOKING TIME: **NONE**

BASE

¼ cup almonds

¼ cup rolled oats

2 Brazil nuts

1 handful kale

6 pitted dates

½ banana, fresh or
    frozen, ripe

½ teaspoon cinnamon

1 dash nutmeg

1 cup plant-based milk,
    unsweetened

TOPPINGS

½ banana, sliced

2 tablespoons chia seeds

2 tablespoons hemp seeds

½ cup berries

1. In a food processor or high-speed blender, add all of the base ingredients and blend until creamy smooth.

2. Divide the base between two bowls.

3. Divide the toppings—sliced banana, chia seeds, hemp seeds, and berries—between the two bowls.

4. Top with more of your favorite topping ingredients and enjoy! Store leftover smoothie base (without the toppings) in the refrigerator for up to 2 days. Add more water or milk as needed to reach the desired consistency.

Per serving: 584 calories, 17 grams protein, 89 grams total carbohydrates (74 grams net carbohydrates), 22.5 grams fat, 15 grams fiber, 70 milligrams sodium

0.75 mcg B12, 425 mg calcium, 6 mg iron, 245 mg magnesium, 103 mcg selenium, 3 mg zinc

---

RECOVERY SMOOTHIE

SERVES: 2 · PREP TIME: **5 MINUTES** · COOKING TIME: **NONE**

½ medium ripe banana, fresh or frozen

½ medium apple

1 ½ cups mixed berries, fresh or frozen

1 handful spinach

1 tablespoon organic peanut butter, unsweetened

2 cups plant-based milk, unsweetened

1 tablespoon chia or hemp seeds

1 handful ice (optional)

1. Place all ingredients in a blender, except the ice and blend until smooth.

2. Check the consistency and add more milk as needed until you reach the desired consistency.

3. Add ice if you like a cool, slushy-style smoothie.

4. Split between two 16-ounce glasses or mason jars. Store leftover smoothie in the refrigerator for up to 2 days. Add more water or milk as needed to reach the desired consistency.

Per serving: 243 calories, 9.5 grams protein, 37 grams total carbohydrates (30 grams net carbohydrates), 9 grams fat, 7 grams fiber, 81 milligrams sodium

1.5 mcg B12, 184 mg calcium, 2 mg iron, 105 mg magnesium, 5.5 mcg selenium, 1.3 mg zinc

PEANUTTY PROTEIN MILKSHAKE

2 cups plant-based milk, unsweetened

¼ cup peanut butter

2 small ripe bananas, fresh or frozen

2 tablespoons hemp seeds, hulled

2 teaspoons vanilla extract

1 teaspoon ground cinnamon

1. Add everything to a high-speed blender. Blend until creamy and smooth.

2. Taste for additional ingredients of choice.

3. Split between two 16-ounce glasses or mason jars.

4. Top with an additional sprinkle of cinnamon. Store leftover smoothie in the refrigerator for up to 2 days. Add more water or milk as needed to reach the desired consistency.

Per serving: 410 calories, 20 grams protein, 35.5 grams total carbohydrates (26.5 grams net carbohydrates), 25 grams fat, 9 grams fiber, 186 milligrams sodium

3 mcg B12, 343 mg calcium, 2.7 mg iron, 195 mg magnesium, 12 mcg selenium, 2.5 mg zinc

REST AND RECOVERY SALADS

I love a good salad. By good I mean, PACKED. A good salad should not just have lettuce. It should be as satisfying as the piled high veggie burger or a big grain bowl. Salads can even be a great recovery meal if you load them up with whole grains and your favorite protein. The salads to follow have tons of colors, which means they are full of nourishment as well as flavors and textures galore.

SUPERFOOD EXTRAVAGANZA SALAD

SERVES: **2** · PREP TIME: **15 MINUTES** · COOKING TIME: **NONE**

3 cups chopped kale leaves

1 cup organic edamame, frozen, thawed

1 cup cooked whole grains, your choice (quinoa, rice, buckwheat, barley, etc.)

1 avocado, cut into cubes

½ cup chopped red onion

½ cup shredded carrots

4 radishes, sliced

2 tablespoons chopped walnuts

2 tablespoons sunflower seeds

2 tablespoons dried cranberries

2 tablespoons hemp seeds

¼ cup chopped herbs (cilantro, basil, or parsley)

1 tablespoon olive oil

Squeeze of lemon

Salt and pepper, to taste

1. To a large bowl, add all ingredients, except olive oil, lemon, salt and pepper, and mix well.

2. Divide between two medium bowls.

3. Drizzle with olive oil, lemon, and taste for salt and pepper. Store leftovers in the refrigerator for up to 3 days.

Per serving: 697 calories, 21.5 grams protein, 65 grams total carbohydrates (45 grams net carbohydrates), 42 grams fat, 20 grams fiber, 61 milligrams sodium

0.0 mcg B12, 231 mg calcium, 6 mg iron, 278 mg magnesium, 13 mcg selenium, 4.4 mg zinc

GLYCOGEN-RESTORING BLACK RICE SALAD

SERVES: **4** · PREP TIME: **20 MINUTES** · COOKING TIME: **NONE**

DRESSING

3 tablespoons rice vinegar

1 tablespoon miso, mellow white or chickpea

1 tablespoon maple syrup

2 tablespoons organic reduced sodium tamari or coconut aminos

1 tablespoon lime juice

1 tablespoon minced ginger

1 tablespoon minced garlic

1 teaspoon red pepper chili flakes (optional)

1 teaspoon toasted sesame oil

3 cups cooked black (or brown) rice

1 cup shredded carrots

1 cup shredded purple cabbage

⅓ cup green onion, sliced

¼ cup chopped cilantro (optional)

2 tablespoons sesame seeds, white or black

¼ cup pumpkin or sunflower seeds

1. To prepare the dressing, whisk together vinegar, miso, maple syrup, tamari, lime juice, ginger, garlic, red pepper chili flakes and sesame seed oil.

2. In a large bowl, add the cooked black rice, carrots, cabbage, and green onions.

3. Add the dressing and toss to combine.

4. Sprinkle cilantro, sesame seeds, and pumpkin or sunflower seeds over top then toss once more before serving. Store leftovers in the refrigerator for up to 5 days.

Per serving (without dressing): 420 calories, 11 grams protein, 72. 5 grams total carbohydrates (67 grams net carbohydrates), 10 grams fat, 6.5 grams fiber, 500 milligrams sodium

0.0 mcg B12, 40 mg calcium, 1.4 mg iron, 55 mg magnesium, 3.6 mcg selenium, 1.1 mg zinc

PLANT-PROTEIN POWERED SALAD

SERVES: **2** · PREP TIME: **10 MINUTES** · COOKING TIME: **NONE**

---

4 packed cups chopped kale

1 tablespoon olive oil

2 cups cooked buckwheat

1½ cups cooked chickpeas

1 large avocado, cubed

1 cup pickled beets

¼ cup chopped walnuts

2–4 tablespoons lemon juice

Salt and pepper, to taste

1. Add the kale to a large bowl. Add the oil and massage it into the kale until the kale becomes tender, about 30 seconds.

2. Add the buckwheat, chickpeas, chopped avocado, pickled beets, and walnuts. Toss to combine.

3. Squeeze the lemon juice on top and sprinkle with salt and pepper. Toss again. Store leftovers in the refrigerator for up to 3 days. Kale is one leafy green that holds up well after being dressed.

4. To make 2 cups buckwheat: Add ½ cup dry rinsed buckwheat to 1 cup boiling water on the stovetop. Reduce heat to low, cover, and cook for 15 minutes. Let rest, covered, for 10 minutes before fluffing with a fork.

Per serving: 720 calories, 18 grams protein, 88 gram total carbohydrates (62 grams net carbohydrates), 36 grams fat, 25 grams fiber, 334 milligrams sodium

0.0 mcg B12, 216 mg calcium, 3.9 mg iron, 203 mg magnesium, 6.5 mcg selenium, 3.2 mg zinc

Main Dishes and Recovery Meals

These recipes are meant to be your day before competition or post-recovery meals where fueling or refueling is warranted. From Ironman Mac 'n Cheese to Champion Chili, these meals are also perfect for the entire family given their size and flavors to satisfy the masses. The veggie burgers are easy to make and perfect for leftovers. Also, you can layer so much goodness on top of burgers. Finally, whenever someone asks me, "What's the best tip for someone who has no time to prepare plant-based meals?" My answer is always bowls. Assembling a bowl when you have the ingredients on hand is an easy and tasty way to pack in a ton of nutrition, flavor, and textures into one meal. Add your sauce or dressing then toss and you are ready to rock and roll. Hope you enjoy these mains as much as I do!

IRONMAN MAC 'N CHEESE

SERVES: 4 · PREP TIME: 10 MINUTES · COOKING TIME: 30 MINUTES

8 ounces whole grain or legume elbow macaroni

1 cups raw cashews, soaked in hot water for 30 minutes, then drained

2 cups plant-based milk, plain & unsweetened

1 cup water

2 tablespoons miso, mellow white or chickpea

5 tablespoons nutritional yeast

2 tablespoons apple cider vinegar

2 tablespoons arrowroot powder or cornstarch

1 teaspoon onion powder

1 teaspoon garlic powder

1 teaspoon ground turmeric

½ teaspoon salt

2 cups broccoli florets cut into 1-inch pieces

1. Make the pasta according to instructions then set it aside.

2. Preheat the oven to 350°F.

3. Make the cashew cheese: Add the cashews, plant-based milk, water, miso, nutritional yeast, apple cider vinegar, arrowroot powder, onion powder, garlic powder, ground turmeric, and salt, if using, to a high-speed blender and blend until smooth. Note that it will be very runny. You are about to thicken it on the stovetop.

4. Transfer the cheese to a large stovetop pot. Add the broccoli and heat over medium-high heat just until it comes to a boil.

5. Reduce heat to medium for a simmer, stirring often (to prevent it from sticking to the bottom of the pan) until the cheese thickens, about 5 minutes.

6. Stir the cooked macaroni into the cashew cheese mixture. Mix until the cheese coats the macaroni.

7. Transfer the Broccoli Mac 'n Cheese to an 8x8" or similar baking dish and bake for 25 minutes.

8. Remove from the oven and let sit for 10–15 minutes. The cheese will further set during this time. Store leftovers in the refrigerator for up to 5 days or in the freezer for up to 30 days.

Per serving: 487 calories, 29 grams protein, 57 grams total carbohydrates (45 grams net carbohydrates), 20 grams fat, 12 grams fiber, 451 milligrams sodium (omit or reduce salt for less sodium)

5.5 mcg B12, 235 mg calcium, 8 mg iron, 198 mg magnesium, 22 mcg selenium, 4 mg zinc

CARB LOADING SPAGHETTI AND "MEATBALLS"

SERVES: **2** · PREP TIME: **40 MINUTES** · COOKING TIME: **30 MINUTES**

8–10 lentil quinoa meatballs, see page 192
8 ounce whole grain or legume spaghetti
Basic Red Tomato Sauce:
1 tablespoon oil
¾ cup chopped white onion
5 large garlic cloves, minced
½ teaspoon red pepper flakes (optional)
½ cup vegetable broth
5 cups chopped tomatoes
1 tablespoon sherry vinegar (or red wine vinegar)
2 tablespoons chopped basil
Salt and pepper, to taste

1. Make ahead of time: Make the Lentil Quinoa Meatballs and keep in the refrigerator for up to 7 days or in the freezer for 30 days. Make sure to thaw them before making this recipe.

2. Make your pasta according to the package instructions. Set aside.

3. Make the Basic Red Tomato Sauce: Heat a large stovetop pan over medium-high heat. Once the pan is hot enough, add the oil and onions. Cook until the onions become translucent, about 3 minutes.

4. Add the garlic and red pepper flakes, if using, and cook for 30 seconds.

5. Add the vegetable stock to deglaze the pan and cook for another minute.

6. Stir in the tomatoes and sherry vinegar and cook on low-medium heat for 20 minutes, continuing to stir occasionally.

7. Add salt and ground black pepper to taste, stir in the basil, then remove from heat. Set aside.

8. In a large stovetop oiled pan, heat 8–10 "meatballs" over medium heat. Cook for 3–5 minutes until browned and warmed through.

9. Add the pasta to a large bowl. Toss in the tomato sauce.

10. Add 4–5 Lentil Quinoa Meatballs to each pasta dish. Store leftover quinoa spaghetti and meatballs in the refrigerator for up to 5 days.

Per serving: Calories: 511 calories, 17 grams protein, 76 grams total carbohydrates (63 grams net carbohydrates), 18 grams fat, 13 grams fiber, 1097 milligrams sodium (omit or reduce salt for less sodium)
2 mcg B12, 79 mg calcium, 6 mg iron, 115 mg magnesium, 20 mcg selenium, 2.7 mg zinc

PLANT-POWERED PR MEATBALLS

SERVES: 4 · PREP TIME: 20 MINUTES · COOKING TIME: 30 MINUTES

1 tablespoon oil

1 cup chopped onion

4 garlic cloves, minced

1 cup grated yellow squash

1 cup chopped spinach

½ cup raw sunflower seeds

1 cup cooked green or brown lentils

2 teaspoons dried oregano

2 tablespoons chopped fresh basil

2 tablespoons nutritional yeast

¼ cup chopped kalamata olives

1 cup cooked quinoa

½ teaspoon red pepper flakes (optional)

½ teaspoon salt

¼ teaspoon pepper

1. Preheat oven to 350°F. Line a baking sheet with parchment paper.

2. Heat the oil in a medium stovetop pan on medium heat. Add the onions and cook until translucent, about 3 minutes.

3. Stir in the garlic and squash and cook for 1–2 minutes.

4. Mix in the spinach until tender. Remove from heat and set aside.

5. In a food processor, coarsely grind the sunflower seeds.

6. Add the onion squash mixture, half of the lentils (½ cup), oregano, basil, nutritional yeast, and olives. Blend until the mixture is smooth.

7. Transfer to a large bowl. Mix in the other ½ cup lentils, quinoa, salt, pepper, and red pepper flakes, if using.

8. Scoop the mixture with a spoon into your hands and roll to form a "meatball" about 1 ½" in diameter.

9. Place the meatballs on the parchment-lined baking sheet. You'll get about 30 small meatballs.

10. Bake for 30 minutes or until crispy on the outside and soft in the middle.

11. Serve with your favorite tomato sauce or with the Quinoa Spaghetti and Meatballs on page 191. Store leftovers in the refrigerator for up to 5 days or freeze for up to 3 months.

Per serving: 228 calories, 11 grams protein, 17 grams total carbohydrates (10.5 grams net carbohydrates), 14 grams fat, 6.5 grams fiber, 285 milligrams sodium (omit or reduce salt for less sodium)

2 mcg B12, 49 mg calcium, 3.2 mg iron, 95 mg magnesium, 16.5 mcg selenium, 2.5 mg zinc

CHAMPION CHILI

1 tablespoon oil
1 cup chopped red onion
1 cup chopped bell pepper
1 large carrot, chopped
8 ounces organic tempeh, crumbled
4 large garlic cloves, minced
2 jalapeño peppers, seeded and diced (optional)
1 tablespoon chili powder
1 tablespoon ground cumin
1 teaspoon onion powder
1 teaspoon garlic powder
1 teaspoon chipotle chili powder (optional)
½ teaspoon salt
¼ teaspoon pepper
1 (28-ounce) can diced tomatoes
3 cups cooked beans (black, kidney, and pinto are great choices)
2 cups vegetable broth
2 cups chopped spinach
¼ cup chopped cilantro (optional)
¼ cup sliced green onion

1. Heat a large soup pot on medium-high heat. Add the oil, onions, carrots, peppers, and tempeh. Cook until the onions are translucent, and tempeh is slightly browned, about 3–4 minutes.

2. Stir in the garlic and cook for another minute.

3. Stir in the spices, salt, and pepper, and jalapeño pepper, if using. Mix well.

4. Add the diced tomatoes, beans and the two cups of vegetable broth. Stir well.

5. Simmer on low for 45–60 minutes (longer for thicker consistency and more concentrated flavors).

6. Remove from heat and stir in the two cups of spinach until tender.

7. Divide between bowls and top with optional cilantro and green onion. Store leftovers in the refrigerator for up to 7 days or in the freezer for up to 3 months.

Per serving: 344 calories, 23 grams protein, 50 grams total carbohydrates (35 grams net carbohydrates), 7 grams fat, 15 grams fiber, 939 milligrams sodium (omit or reduce salt for less sodium)

Trace amounts B12, 172 mg calcium, 4.7 mg iron, 120 mg magnesium, 3.7 mcg selenium, 2.2 mg zinc

RUNNER'S HIGH RAMEN

SERVES: 2 · PREP TIME: 15 MINUTES · COOKING TIME: 20 MINUTES

1 tablespoon oil
2 cups chopped mushrooms
1 cup chopped onion
1 cup chopped red bell pepper
1 bunch bok choy, stems and leaves
    chopped and separated
1 tablespoon grated garlic cloves
1 tablespoon grated fresh ginger
1 tablespoon grated fresh lemongrass
4 cups vegetable broth
2 cups water
8 ounces brown rice noodles
2 tablespoons miso

2–3 teaspoons gochujang or other
    chili paste
1 cup light coconut milk
2 tablespoons organic reduced-sodium
    tamari or coconut aminos
1 cup organic frozen shelled edamame,
    thawed
2 tablespoons lime juice
2 green onions, white and green parts,
    thinly sliced
chopped cilantro to taste (optional)
Sriracha to taste (optional)

1. Heat a large stockpot on medium-high heat. Add the oil, mushrooms, onion, red pepper, and bok choy stems, stirring occasionally until the onions are translucent, about 3 minutes.

2. Stir in the garlic, ginger, and lemongrass. Cook for another minute.

3. Add the vegetable broth and water. Bring to a boil then add the noodles.

4. Continue to boil and cook the noodles for 10 minutes or until tender.

5. In a medium bowl, combine miso, coconut milk, tamari, and gochujang. Whisk until miso is completely dissolved.

6. Once the noodles are tender, turn off the heat and transfer the coconut milk mixture to the veggie ramen and stir.

7. Add the bok choy leaves and edamame, stirring until the bok choy leaves are tender. Squeeze in the lime juice.

8. Divide the ramen between four bowls and garnish with a generous amount of green onion, cilantro, and sriracha, if using. Best if consumed immediately. If planning to make extra for leftovers then cook and store the noodles separately and add when you're ready to reheat the broth.

Per serving: 360 calories, 18 grams protein, 68.5 grams total carbohydrates (50 grams net carbohydrates), 7 grams fat, 8.5 grams fiber, 1375 milligrams sodium (use coconut aminos for less sodium)

Trace amounts B12, 97 mg calcium, 4.5 mg iron, 53 mg magnesium, 5.7 mcg selenium, 1.2 mg zinc

STAMINA BEET BURGERS

¾ cup sunflower seeds

¼ cup flax meal

3 medium garlic cloves

1½ tablespoons miso, mellow white or chickpea

1 tablespoon chili powder

1 tablespoon cumin powder

1 teaspoon ground turmeric

1 tablespoon onion powder

½ teaspoon salt

⅛ teaspoon pepper

1 cup grated beets (scrub well and leave skin on)

1 cup rolled oats

1½ cups cooked white beans

1–2 medium pitted avocados, flesh removed and smashed with a fork

PICKLED RED ONIONS

½ medium red onion, thinly sliced

½ cup red wine vinegar

½ cup water

¼ teaspoon salt

Organic whole grain bread

1. Preheat the oven to 375°F. Line a baking sheet with parchment paper.

2. Add the sunflower seeds, flax meal, garlic cloves, miso, chili powder, cumin, turmeric, onion powder, and salt and pepper to a food processor. Blend until a moist coarse dough forms.

3. Add the beets, oats, and beans. Blend until combined, using a spatula to scrape the sides and bottom of the food processor, making sure that everything is blended.

4. With clean hands, scoop out the burger mix to form 4-inch patties about ½-inch thick. You should get about 6 thick patties.

5. Bake for 40 minutes, flipping halfway through.

6. Meanwhile, make your pickled red onions: Add the onions, vinegar, water, and salt to a medium bowl. Massage the onions with your hands for 30–60 seconds. Set aside.

7. Once the burgers are done, top with smashed avocado and pickled red onions and enjoy as is or in between whole-grain bread with more of your favorite fixings. Store leftovers in the refrigerator for 5–7 days or freeze, separating each burger with parchment paper and placing in a freezer-safe container, for up to 30 days.

Per patty (bun and toppings not included): 258 calories, 9 grams protein, 25 grams total carbohydrates (17 grams net carbohydrates), 15 grams fat, 8 grams fiber, 285 milligrams sodium

0.0 mcg B12, 60 mg calcium, 3.2 mg iron, 101 mg magnesium, 14 mcg selenium, 1.8 mg zinc

CROSS COUNTRY LENTIL BURGERS

SERVES: **6** • PREP TIME: **30** • COOKING TIME: **45**

1 cup dry lentils, brown
    or green
3 cups + 4 tablespoons water
2 tablespoons flax meal
½ cup raw walnuts
1 tablespoon dried oregano
¾ cup rolled oats
1 tablespoon oil
1 cup diced carrots
1 cup diced yellow onion
4 garlic cloves, minced
2 tablespoons tomato paste
2 tablespoons vegan
    Worcestershire sauce
1 tablespoon organic
    reduced-sodium tamari or
    coconut aminos
½ cup organic oat flour
¼ teaspoon salt
¼ teaspoon pepper

1. Rinse the lentils well then place in a medium stovetop pot. Add 3 cups of water. Bring to a high simmer then lower the heat. Cover and cook for 25 minutes or until tender (almost to the mushy stage works well for these burgers).

2. In the meantime, add the flax meal and 4 tablespoons of water to a small bowl and let sit. This will be your "flax egg," which binds the burgers.

3. Place the walnuts, oats, and oregano in a food processor. Blend until the walnuts and oats are coarsely blended. Set aside.

4. Heat a stovetop pan on medium-high heat. Add the oil, carrots, onions, and garlic. Cook for 5–7 minutes, stirring occasionally until the carrots are tender.

5. Lower the heat, add the tomato paste, Worcestershire sauce, and tamari. With a spatula, mix until the sauce is combined with the carrot, onion and garlic mixture.

6. In a large bowl, add ½ of the cooked lentils from the pot and mash with a fork or potato masher.

7. Add the remaining lentils (so half of the lentils will be mashed, and half will be whole).

8. Mix in the carrot, onion and garlic mixture; the oats and walnuts mixture; and the oat flour, salt, and pepper. Mix until all ingredients are combined.

9. Fold in the flax egg.

10. Form eight individual patties with your hands and place on a clean cutting board.

THE VEGAN ATHLETE'S NUTRITION HANDBOOK

11. Heat a stovetop pan or griddle that is lightly oiled over medium heat. Once the skillet is nice and hot, cook the burgers on each side until browned for about 5 minutes per side. Store leftovers in the refrigerator for 5–7 days or freeze, separating each burger with parchment paper and placing in a freezer-safe container, for up to 30 days.

Per patty (bun and toppings not included): 214 calories, 9 grams protein, 28 grams total carbohydrates (21 grams net carbohydrates), 8.5 grams fat, 7 grams fiber, 393 milligrams sodium

0.0 mcg B12, 72 mg calcium, 3.5 mg iron, 67 mg magnesium, 8 mcg selenium, 1.6 mg zinc

THE ULTIMATE RECOVERY PURPLE-POWERED BOWL

SERVES: 2 · PREP TIME: 20 MINUTES · COOKING TIME: 40 MINUTES

ROASTED CHICKPEAS AND VEGETABLES

1½ cups cooked chickpeas
¼ teaspoon salt
¼ teaspoon ground black pepper
2 cups purple potatoes, washed, cut into 1-inch cubes (skin on)
2 small beets, scrubbed, greens removed, cut into 1-inch cubes (skin on or off)
1–2 tablespoons oil

BOWL INGREDIENTS

4 cups organic kale leaves, sliced into ribbons
½ small red onion, thinly sliced on a mandoline or manually with a knife
1 cup red cabbage, shredded
1 batch Breakaway Blueberry Dressing, see page 207

1. Preheat the oven to 400°F, and line a baking sheet with parchment paper.

2. Spread the chickpeas on one side and the potatoes on the other side of the baking sheet. Spread each of them out evenly. Drizzle with a little oil and sprinkle with salt and pepper.

3. Place the beets in parchment paper (enough to wrap around them). Place foil around the parchment paper and bring the edges of the foil up to seal for steaming the beets. Place on a small baking sheet.

4. Roast the chickpeas, potatoes, and beets for 35–40 minutes (or until the chickpeas are crispy and potatoes and beets are tender), tossing the chickpeas and potatoes halfway through. Remove from the oven, and set aside.

5. Meanwhile, prepare your bowl ingredients: Divide the kale, onion, cabbage between two bowls.

6. When the beets, potatoes, and chickpeas are finished cooking, divide them between the two bowls.

7. Divide the Breakaway Blueberry Dressing to each bowl.

8. Top with freshly ground pepper and more salt, if desired. Store leftovers in the refrigerator for up to 5 days.

Per serving: 529 calories, 20 grams protein, 104 grams total carbohydrates (84 grams net carbohydrates), 4 grams fat, 20 grams fiber, 809 milligrams sodium

0.0 mcg B12, 290 mg calcium, 9 mg iron, 200 mg magnesium, 7.2 mcg selenium, 4.2 mg zinc

LOADED LENTIL AND CORN MEXICAN BOWL

SERVES: 4 · PREP TIME: 15 MINUTES · COOKING TIME: 30 MINUTES

4 cups cubed sweet potatoes, washed and cut into 1-inch cubes
1 tablespoon oil

MEXICAN SEASONING
½ teaspoon onion powder
½ teaspoon garlic powder
½ teaspoon paprika
¼ teaspoon chili powder
1 teaspoon ground cumin
½ teaspoon salt
¼ teaspoon ground black pepper

LENTILS AND CORN
2 cups cooked lentils brown or green
2 cups organic corn, frozen or cooked from fresh
2 tablespoons lime juice

KALE
4 cups chopped kale leaves
1 teaspoon oil
2 tablespoons lemon juice
Salt, to taste

TOPPINGS
½ cup red onion, diced
½ cup purple cabbage, shredded
2–4 tablespoons diced jalapeño (seeded)
1 large avocado, cubed
2–4 tablespoons cilantro, chopped (optional)
Cashew Cheese Sauce (optional), see page 190

1. Preheat oven to 400°F and line a baking sheet with parchment paper.

2. Mix the seasoning ingredients together in a small bowl.

3. Add the sweet potatoes to a large bowl. Toss in the oil, half of the seasoning and stir to coat the sweet potatoes. (Save the other half of the seasoning.)

4. Spread the sweet potatoes out evenly on the parchment-lined baking sheet and bake for 30 minutes, tossing halfway through.

5. Make the lentils and corn: Add the cooked lentils and corn to a large bowl. Add the lime juice and remaining spice blend. Mix well to coat the lentils and corn with the lime and spices. Set aside.

6. Add the kale to a large bowl. Add the oil, lemon juice and a sprinkle of salt. Massage the kale until tender, about 30 seconds.

7. Split the kale, the lentil and corn mixture and sweet potatoes between four bowls.

8. Divide the onion, cabbage and jalapeño on top of each bowl.

9. Top with avocado cubes. Sprinkle with cilantro, if using.

10. Squeeze more lime or drizzle Cashew Cheese Sauce over top. Store leftovers in the refrigerator for up to 5 days.

Per serving: 408 calories, 16 grams protein, 75 grams total carbohydrates (58 grams net carbohydrates), 7 grams fat, 17 grams fiber, 485 milligrams sodium

0.0 mcg B12, 158 mg calcium, 5.5 mg iron, 116 mg magnesium, 4 mcg selenium, 2.5 mg zinc

LONG, SLOW AND STEADY TEMPEH FARRO BOWL

SERVES: 4 • PREP TIME: 20 MINUTES • COOKING TIME: 25 MINUTES

CASHEW CHEESE SAUCE

1 cup cashews, soaked in hot water for
    30 minutes, drained

2 tablespoons lemon juice

½ cup water

1 tablespoon apple cider vinegar

¼ teaspoon salt

½ teaspoon onion powder

TEMPEH

8 ounce organic tempeh, cut in half so
    you have two pieces

1 tablespoon oil

1 cup chopped white onion

3 large garlic cloves, minced

½ teaspoon red pepper flakes (optional)

½ cup vegetable broth

4 cups tomatoes, chopped

2 tablespoons tomato paste

1 tablespoon sherry vinegar (or red wine
    vinegar)

2 teaspoons dried oregano

¼ teaspoon salt

¼ ground black pepper

2 tablespoons chopped basil or parsley,
    chopped

2 cups chopped spinach

¼ cup diced green olives

¼ cup diced artichoke hearts

4 cups cooked farro (or other grain of
    choice)

1. Make the cashew cheese: Add all ingredients to a food processor or blender and blend until smooth. Taste for additional flavors of your choice. Set aside.

2. Boil the tempeh: In a medium stovetop pot, add enough water to cover the tempeh and bring to a boil. Add the tempeh.

3. Boil for 10 minutes. When done, remove from the water. Once cool, crumble the tempeh into bite-sized pieces into a bowl. Set aside.

4. Make the tomato sauce and tempeh: Heat a large stovetop pan on medium/high. Add the oil and onions, cooking the onions until translucent, about 3 minutes.

5. Add the garlic and cook for 30 seconds. Stir in the chili flakes, if using.

6. Add the vegetable broth, tomatoes, crumbled tempeh, tomato paste, sherry vinegar, and oregano. Stir well and cook on low-medium heat for 20 minutes, stirring occasionally.

7. Add salt and ground black pepper then remove from heat.

8. Lastly, stir in the basil (or parsley) and spinach and stir until they're tender.

9. Divide the cooked farro between two bowls.

10. Add 1 cup of the tomato tempeh mixture to each bowl.

11. Garnish with olives and artichokes.

12. Top with 3–4 tablespoons cashew cheese. Store leftovers in the refrigerator for up to 5 days.

Per serving: 577 calories, 27 grams protein, 67 grams total carbohydrates (55 grams net carbohydrates), 27 grams fat, 12 grams fiber, 617 milligrams sodium

Trace amounts B12, 143 mg calcium, 6.5 mg iron, 252 mg magnesium, 44 mcg selenium, 4.7 mg zinc

Dressings

Here you will find some of my personal favorite sauces and dressings. To make healthy meal prep super easy, I love to keep 2–3 sauces or dressings in my fridge at all times since they can instantly elevate salads, wraps and grain bowls. What is cool about the sauces and dressings is that, since they are made with whole food ingredients like tofu, nuts, and seeds, they also have some protein and fiber (something you cannot find in most store-bought dressings and sauces).

GREEN GODDESS DRESSING

SERVES: **4** · PREP TIME: **10 MINUTES** · COOKING TIME: **NONE**

¼ cup tahini

5 tablespoons water

1 medium lemon, juiced

1 tablespoon apple cider
   vinegar

1 tablespoon maple syrup

1 small garlic clove, chopped

1 stalk green onion, chopped,
   including the white and
   green portions

½ cup cilantro, chopped
   (substitute basil or parsley
   if cilantro is not your
   thing!)

1. Add all ingredients to a blender or food processor and blend until creamy.

2. Add more water, 1 tablespoon at a time, if
needed for desired consistency. Store in the refrigerator for up to 7 days.

Per serving: 108 calories, 2.5 grams protein, 7.5 grams total
carbohydrates (6 grams net carbohydrates), 8 grams fat, 1.5 grams fiber,
20 milligrams sodium

0.0 mcg B12, 75 mg calcium, 1.4 mg iron, 17 mg magnesium, 5 mcg selenium,
0.8 mg zinc

10/10 PEANUT SAUCE

SERVES: **4** · PREP TIME: **5 MINUTES** · COOKING TIME: **NONE**

1 tablespoon miso, mellow white or chickpea

¼ cup unsweetened peanut butter

2 tablespoons organic reduced-sodium tamari or coconut aminos

1 tablespoon rice vinegar

1 tablespoon maple syrup

1–2 teaspoons chili paste or other hot sauce of choice (optional)

2 teaspoons grated ginger

1 teaspoon grated garlic

¼ cup water

1. Place all ingredients in a medium bowl and whisk until the peanut butter and miso are completely dissolved. Alternatively, you could add all ingredients to a high-speed blender and blend until smooth.

2. Taste for additional ingredients of choice (ginger for spice, tamari for umami, peanut butter for peanut). Store in the refrigerator for up to 7 days. Note, it may thicken as it sits. Add 1–2 tablespoons of water to return it to a sauce consistency.

Per serving: Calories: 122 calories, 5 grams protein, 8.5 grams total carbohydrates (7.5 grams net carbohydrates), 8 grams fat, 1 gram fiber, 431 milligrams sodium

0.0 mcg B12, 17 mg calcium, 0.5 mg iron, 33 mg magnesium, 1 mcg selenium, 0.5 mg zinc

ULTRA LEMON DIJON DRESSING

SERVES: **4** · PREP TIME: **5 MINUTES** · COOKING TIME: **NONE**

1 cup plant-based yogurt, unsweetened
1 tablespoon tahini
1 tablespoon Dijon mustard
2 tablespoons lemon juice
2 tablespoons apple cider vinegar
2 tablespoons roughly chopped shallots
1 tablespoon maple syrup
¼ teaspoon salt

1. Add all ingredients to a blender or food processor and blend until creamy.

2. Taste for additional flavors (more lemon for acidity, more yogurt for tang, more Dijon for Dijon!).

3. Use on salads, grain bowls, or as a veggie dip. Store in the refrigerator for up to 5 days.

Per serving: 102 calories, 1 gram protein, 18 grams total carbohydrates (16 grams net carbohydrates), 3.5 grams fat, 2 grams fiber, 117 milligrams sodium

0.0 mcg B12, 103 mg calcium, 0.7 mg iron, 17 mg magnesium, 1.5 mcg selenium, 0.4 mg zinc

BREAKAWAY BLUEBERRY DRESSING

SERVES: 4 · PREP TIME: 5 MINUTES · COOKING TIME: NONE

1 cup blueberries, fresh or
   frozen
¼ cup water
2 tablespoons tahini
2 tablespoons balsamic
   vinegar
2–3 tablespoons maple
   syrup
1½ teaspoons Dijon
   mustard
2 tablespoons lime juice
Salt, to taste
Ground black pepper,
   to taste

1. Add all ingredients to a blender or food processor and blend until smooth.

2. Taste and adjust as needed (more water for consistency, maple for sweetness or to offset acidity, or blueberries for more berry flavor). Store in the refrigerator for up to 5 days.

Per serving: 103 calories, 1.5 grams protein, 15.5 grams total carbohydrates (14 grams net carbohydrates), 4 grams fat, 1.5 grams fiber, 57 milligrams sodium

0.0 mcg B12, 49 mg calcium, 0.8 mg iron, 14 mg magnesium, 3 mcg selenium, 0.7 mg zinc

Stamina-Building Snacks

Whether you are looking for an everyday snack to satisfy your crunchy cravings or a snack to keep you fueled and energized, you will find at least one (hopefully more!) here. All of these snacks take less than 15 minutes to prepare (many only take 5 minutes to prep!), therefore, I would suggest making one or two for the week so you have them for fuel throughout the day or during your training. A key component to good nutrition and staying fueled is having whole, unprocessed food ready-to-go whenever you need it.

ENDURANCE BANANA BREAD

PLANT-BASED BUTTERMILK

¼ cup plant-based milk, unsweetened (soy seems to work best!)

2 teaspoons apple cider vinegar

DRY INGREDIENTS

2 cups oat flour

1 teaspoon baking soda

¾ teaspoon baking powder

¾ teaspoon cinnamon

½ teaspoon salt

WET INGREDIENTS

1½ cups mashed banana (about 3 medium ripe bananas)

¼ cup maple syrup

2 teaspoons vanilla extract

¾ cup walnuts, chopped

1. Preheat the oven to 350°F. Prepare a 9x5-inch loaf pan (or similar size) by lining it with parchment paper or spraying it with oil.

2. Make the buttermilk: In a small bowl, add the milk and the apple cider vinegar. Stir then set aside while you prepare the remaining ingredients.

3. Add the dry ingredients to a large bowl and stir. Set aside.

4. Mix the mashed banana, maple syrup, and vanilla together in a medium bowl.

5. Pour the wet ingredients into the large mixing bowl with the dry ingredients. Add the buttermilk and stir. Don't overmix! A little lumpiness is okay.

6. Stir in the walnuts (omit for nut-free).

7. Pour the batter into the baking dish and bake for 45 minutes or until browned on top and cooked through the center (baking time may vary depending on your oven).

8. Store in the refrigerator for up to 5 days. To store in the freezer, slice the bread into individual pieces and wrap them separately in parchment paper before storing in the freezer for up to 30 days.

Per serving: 335 calories, 8 grams protein, 51 grams total carbohydrates (44 grams net carbohydrates), 12.5 grams fat, 7 grams fiber, 205 milligrams sodium

0.1 mcg B12, 67 mg calcium, 2.3 mg iron, 98 mg magnesium, 13 mcg selenium, 2.2 mg zinc

NO-BAKE NUTTY SEEDY BARS

SERVES: 8 · PREP TIME: **5 MINUTES** · COOKING TIME: **NONE**

1 cup pitted dates
¼ cup chia seeds
½ cup shredded coconut, unsweetened
1 cup chopped walnuts
1 cup chopped pecans
½ cup rolled oats
1 teaspoon vanilla extract
½ teaspoon ground cinnamon
2 pinches salt

1. Add all ingredients to a food processor and blend until a moist, thick dough forms.

2. Line a square baking dish with parchment paper. Firmly press the mixture into the dish, making sure it is tight in all corners.

3. Place in the freezer for a few hours up to overnight.

4. Lift out of the dish from the parchment paper onto a cutting board and cut into 8 bars. Store in in the refrigerator for up to 10 days or freezer for up to one month.

Per serving: 305 calories, 7 grams protein, 20.5 grams total carbohydrates (14 grams net carbohydrates), 24 grams fat, 6.5 grams fiber, 40 milligrams sodium

0.0 mcg B12, 65 mg calcium, 2 mg iron, 77 mg magnesium, 6.7 mcg selenium, 1.6 mg zinc

CHOCOLATE CHIP BLONDIES

2 cups rolled oats
1 medium ripe banana
¼ cup almond butter
4 pitted dates
1 teaspoon vanilla extract
½ cup shredded coconut, unsweetened
1 pinch salt
¼ cup vegan chocolate chips, fair trade

1. In a food processor, blend the oats until they are coarsely ground. Transfer them into a medium bowl and set aside.

2. Add the banana, almond butter, dates, vanilla extract, and salt to the food processor.

3. Blend until smooth.

4. Scoop banana mixture into the medium bowl with the coarsely ground oats.

5. Mix until a moist dough is formed.

6. Mix in the shredded coconut and chocolate chips, if using.

7. Add the mixture to a parchment-lined square or rectangular dish. With a spatula or your hands, press the mixture firmly into the dish to the corners.

8. Freeze for 1–2 hours.

9. Pull from the freezer, pull out the parchment paper and dough. Place on a cutting board and cut into squares or rectangles. Store in the refrigerator for up to 7 days or in the freezer for up to 30 days.

Per serving: 238 calories, 5.5 grams protein, 31.5 grams total carbohydrates (26 grams net carbohydrates), 11 grams fat, 5.5 grams fiber, 20 milligrams sodium

0.0 mcg B12, 51 mg calcium, 2.1 mg iron, 78 mg magnesium, 7.5 mcg selenium, 1.4 mg zinc

FINISH LINE COOKIE DOUGH

1½ cups cooked chickpeas

¼ cup almond butter

2–4 tablespoons maple syrup

¼ cup rolled oats

2 teaspoons vanilla extract

½ teaspoon baking soda (only needed if you plan to bake but fine to add it "just in case")

¼ teaspoon salt

⅓ cup vegan chocolate chips, fair trade (optional)

⅓ cup chopped walnuts (optional)

1. Add all ingredients except the vegan chocolate chips and walnuts to a food processor.

2. Blend until creamy smooth.

3. Transfer the cookie dough to a bowl and stir in the chocolate chips and walnuts, if using. Store in the refrigerator for up to 5 days or freeze for up to 30 days.

4. If you plan to bake: Line a baking sheet with parchment paper. Drop rounded tablespoon sizes of batter onto the baking sheet with 2–3 inches between each cookie. Flatten the cookies with a fork (they won't spread much). Bake at 350°F for 12–15 minutes.

Per serving: 239 calories, 7 grams protein, 22.5 grams total carbohydrates (17 grams net carbohydrates), 15 grams fat, 5.5 grams fiber, 205 milligrams sodium

0.0 mcg B12, 74 mg calcium, 2.1 mg iron, 75 mg magnesium, 3.3 mcg selenium, 1.3 mg zinc

COOL DOWN CHIA PUDDING

SERVES: 2 · PREP TIME: 5 MINUTES · COOKING TIME: NONE

PUDDING

1 cup plant-based milk,
   unsweetened
¼ cup chia seeds
½ cup pumpkin puree
2½ tablespoons maple syrup
1 teaspoon vanilla extract
1 teaspoon pumpkin pie
   spice or ground cinnamon

VANILLA CASHEW CREAM

1 cup cashews, soaked in
   hot water for 30 minutes,
   drained
½ cup plant-based milk,
   unsweetened
¼ cup maple syrup
1 teaspoon vanilla extract
1 pinch salt (optional)

1. Add the pudding ingredients (from the plant-based milk to the pumpkin pie spice) to a blender or food processor.

2. Blend until smooth.

3. Transfer the pudding into a bowl (or two individual bowls) and refrigerate for at least four hours.

4. Meanwhile, make the vanilla cashew cream: Add the cashews, plant-based milk, maple, vanilla, and salt into a blender or food processor.

5. Blend until smooth.

6. Top the pudding with one or two dollops of vanilla cashew cream and a sprinkle of cinnamon, if desired. Store in the refrigerator for up to 5 days.

Per serving: 322 calories, 12 grams protein, 37 grams total carbohydrates (26.5 grams net carbohydrates), 16 grams fat, 10.5 grams fiber, 63 milligrams sodium

1.8 mcg B12, 352 mg calcium, 5.6 mg iron, 155 mg magnesium, 18 mcg selenium, 2.6 mg zinc

Tables and References

GRAINS AND NUTRITIONAL CONTENT			
Grain	**Nutrients**	**Fun Fact**	**Gluten free**
Amaranth (Actually, a seed with nutrient composition similar to grains)	Grain highest in protein (9 grams per cooked cup) especially lysine which is not found in most grains; good source of fiber, iron, selenium, B vitamins; excellent source of magnesium, phosphorus, manganese; also has a compound called lunasin that may fight inflammation	Amaranth contains adequate levels of all essential amino acids (also known as a "complete" protein). Amaranth is sold on the streets of South America, popped, like popcorn.	Yes
Barley	Good source of protein, magnesium, phosphorus, niacin (B3) and copper; excellent source of fiber, thiamine, manganese, and selenium	Barley may be even more effective than oats in lowering cholesterol due to its type of fiber (beta glucan).	No
Buckwheat (Relative of rhubarb family with a composition similar to grains)	Good source of protein, fiber, phosphorus, riboflavin (B2), niacin (B3); excellent source of manganese, magnesium, and copper; also has an antioxidant called rutin that's been shown to help with heart health	Similar to amaranth and quinoa, buckwheat has adequate amounts of all essential amino acids (also known as "complete" protein). Buckwheat contains resistant starch which acts as a prebiotic (good for gut health!).	Yes
Bulgur	Good source of protein, iron, magnesium, phosphorus, zinc, riboflavin (B2) and niacin (B3); excellent source of fiber and manganese	Bulgur in the grocery store has been precooked and dried, meaning it only takes 10 minutes for you to prepare (quick-cooking grain!).	No
Corn	Good source of fiber, magnesium, manganese, phosphorus, selenium, thiamine (B1); excellent source of carotenoids lutein and zeaxanthin (important for eye health)	Corn is packed with antioxidants. Choose organic whenever possible since much of the corn in the U.S. is GMO.	Yes

GRAINS AND NUTRITIONAL CONTENT			
Grain	**Nutrients**	**Fun Fact**	**Gluten free**
Einkorn	Good source of protein, iron, magnesium, phosphorus, zinc, riboflavin (B2) and niacin (B3); excellent source of fiber and manganese	Compared to traditional wheat, einkorn has been shown to be higher in protein and carotenoids.	No
Farro	Good source of protein, iron, magnesium, phosphorus, zinc, riboflavin (B2) and niacin (B3); excellent source of fiber and manganese	It is also known as Emmer, an ancient grain that was one of the first cultivated until traditional wheat became available and easier to hull.	No
Freekeh	Good source of protein, iron, magnesium, phosphorus, zinc, riboflavin (B2) and niacin (B3); excellent source of fiber and manganese	It is a hard wheat that is harvested when the plant is still young and green, then roasted and rubbed, giving it a smoky flavor.	No
Kamut	Good source of protein, iron, magnesium, phosphorus, zinc, riboflavin (B2) and niacin (B3); excellent source of fiber and manganese	Compared to traditional wheat, kamut has more protein and vitamin E.	No
Kañiwa (a cousin of quinoa)		Studies show that it is high in the antioxidant quercetin.	Yes
Millet	Good source protein, fiber, magnesium, copper, phosphorus; excellent source of manganese	Millet is extremely versatile and can be used in everything from flatbreads to hot cereal, side dishes and desserts. It is high in protein and antioxidants.	Yes
Oats	Good source of protein, selenium, fiber, iron, thiamine (B1), magnesium, phosphorus, zinc, and copper; excellent source of manganese.	Oats have a prebiotic fiber called beta glucan that has been shown to lower cholesterol; they also have an antioxidant called avenanthramides that are also cardioprotective.	Look for gluten free oats
Quinoa (Not a true grain; relative of beets with a composition similar to grains)	Good source (greater than or equal to 10% of the recommended daily good source of copper, protein, fiber, and iron, thiamine (B1) and pyridoxine (B6); excellent source of magnesium, phosphorus, manganese, and folic acid.	Quinoa has adequate amounts of all essential amino acids (also known as "complete" protein).	Yes

GRAINS AND NUTRITIONAL CONTENT			
Grain	**Nutrients**	**Fun Fact**	**Gluten free**
Rice (brown, black or red)	Good source of fiber, magnesium, phosphorus, selenium, thiamine (B1), niacin (B3) and pyridoxine (B6). Excellent source of manganese.	Black rice is packed with anthocyanins, a phytonutrient that has been shown to help with heart health, brain health and gut health.	Yes
Rye	Good source of magnesium, phosphorus, copper, selenium, and niacin (B3); excellent source of fiber and manganese.	Look for whole rye or rye berries to ensure you are getting the whole grain.	No
Sorghum	Good source of fiber, magnesium, phosphorus, and thiamine (B3); excellent source of manganese.	About half of cultivated sorghum is used for animal feed and to make packaging.	Yes
Spelt	Good source of protein, iron, magnesium, phosphorus, zinc, riboflavin (B2) and niacin (B3); excellent source of fiber and manganese.	The texture is light and airy like wheat flour and can be substituted in baking cakes, cookies, pancakes and bread for a healthy alternative to wheat flour.	No
Teff	Good source of essential fatty acids, fiber, calcium iron, and phytonutrients.	Teff has three times the calcium as other grains. Teff's protein is easily digestible similar to egg whites.	Yes
Triticale	Good source of protein, iron, magnesium, phosphorus, zinc, riboflavin (B2) and niacin (B3); excellent source of fiber and manganese.	It grows easily without commercial fertilizers and pesticides, making it ideal for organic and sustainable farming.	No
Wheat	Good source of protein, iron, magnesium, phosphorus, zinc, riboflavin (B2) and niacin (B3); excellent source of fiber and manganese.	Varieties of wheat include triticale, bulgur, cracked wheat and wheat berries.	No
Wild Rice (actually a member of the grass family with composition similar to wheat)	Higher in protein than most other whole grains; good source of fiber, folate, magnesium, phosphorus, manganese, zinc, pyridoxine (B6), and niacin (B3).	Research shows that antioxidants in wild rice is 30 times greater than that of white rice.	Yes

https://wholegrainscouncil.org/whole-grains-101/whole-grains-z

PROTEIN CONTENT IN PLANT-BASED FOODS

Food	Serving Size	Protein (grams)
Grains		
Amaranth (technically a seed)	1 cup, cooked	9.5
Buckwheat	groats, 1 cup, cooked	6
Chickpea pasta	1 cup, cooked	11
Corn	1 cup	4
Farro	1 cup, cooked	6.5
Lentil pasta	1 cup, cooked	14
Millet	1 cup, cooked	6
Oats	1 cup, cooked	11
Quinoa (technically a seed)	1 cup, cooked	8
Rice, brown	1 cup, cooked	6
Sorghum	¼ cup, dry (yields ¾ cup cooked)	5
Teff	1 cup, cooked	9
Whole grain bread	1 slice	3–5
Whole Wheat pasta	1 cup, cooked	8
Wild Rice (technically a grass)	1 cup, cooked	7
Beans, Peas, and Lentils		
Black beans	1 cup, cooked	14
Cannellini beans	1 cup, cooked	12
Chickpeas	1 cup, cooked	11
Edamame	1 cup, cooked	19
Great Northern beans	1 cup, cooked	17
Kidney beans	1 cup, cooked	14
Lentils	1 cup, cooked	18
Peas	1 cup, cooked	8
Tempeh	3 ounces	23
Tofu	3 ounces	14

PROTEIN CONTENT IN PLANT-BASED FOODS		
Food	**Serving Size**	**Protein (grams)**
Nuts		
Almonds	1 ounce	6
Brazil nuts	1 ounce	4
Cashews	1 ounce	5
Hazelnuts	1 ounce	4
Macadamia nuts	1 ounce	2
Peanuts (technically a legume)	1 ounce	7
Pecans	1 ounce	3
Pistachios	1 ounce	6
Walnuts	1 ounce	4
Seeds		
Chia	2 tablespoons	3
Flax meal	2 tablespoons	3
Hemp	2 tablespoons	13
Pumpkin	2 tablespoons	4.5
Sesame	2 tablespoons	4
Sunflower	2 tablespoons	4
Nut and Seed Butter		
Almond butter	2 tablespoons	7
Cashew butter	2 tablespoons	6
Peanut butter	2 tablespoons	8
Sunflower butter	2 tablespoons	5.5
Tahini	2 tablespoons	5
Plant-Based Milk		
Soy milk	1 cup	8
Hemp milk	1 cup	2
Almond milk	1 cup	1

CALCIUM CONTENT IN PLANT-BASED FOODS		
Food	Serving Size	Calcium Content
Almonds	1 ounce	76 mg
Amaranth	1 cup	116 mg
Broccoli, boiled	1 cup	62 mg
Brussel sprouts	8 sprouts	60 mg
Butternut squash, boiled	1 cup	84 mg
Chia seeds	1 ounce	179 mg
Chickpeas, canned	1 cup	109 mg
Collards, boiled	1 cup	268 mg
Figs, dried	10 medium	175 mg
Great northern beans, boiled	1 cup	120 mg
Kale, boiled	1 cup	177 mg
Mustard greens, boiled	1 cup	165 mg
Navel orange	1 medium	60 mg
Navy beans, boiled	1 cup	128 mg
Orange juice, calcium-fortified	1 cup	349 mg
Pinto beans, boiled	1 cup	79 mg
Tofu	½ cup	160 - 320 mg
Spinach, boiled	1 cup	245 mg
Soybeans, boiled	1 cup	175 mg
Sweet potato, boiled	1 cup	109 mg
Tahini	2 Tablespoons	130 mg
Teff, cooked	1 cup	123 mg

MAGNESIUM CONTENT IN PLANT-BASED FOODS		
Food	**Serving**	**Magnesium**
Almonds	1 ounce	77 mg
Amaranth, cooked	1 cup	174 mg
Avocado	1 medium	58 mg
Beets	1 cup	65 mg
Black beans, cooked	1 cup	120 mg
Brazil nuts	1 ounce	107 mg
Brown rice, cooked	1 cup	79 mg
Buckwheat, flour	½ cup	151 mg
Cannellini beans, cooked	1 cup	120 mg
Cashews	1 ounce	83 mg
Chia seeds	2 tablespoons	78 mg
Dates (Medjool)	3 dates	39 mg
Dark Chocolate	1 ounce	471 mg
Edamame, shelled	1 cup	99 mg
Flaxseeds	2 tablespoons	82 mg
Hemp seeds, hulled	2 tablespoons	140 mg
Lentils, cooked	1 cup	71 mg
Pumpkin seeds	2 tablespoons	100 mg
Quinoa, cooked	1 cup	118 mg
Sunflower seeds	2 tablespoons	57 mg
Teff, flour	½ cup	147 mg
Tempeh	3 ounces	66 mg

Resources and Further Reading

Resources can be very helpful when getting started. Resources are also helpful in staying inspired. Either way, you are covered here. Whether you are vegan or veg-curious for health, the planet, or animals, you should find some great resources below. Being plant-based might seem challenging at times. I hope these resources make it a little easier for you!

Lifestyle Blogs

For those wanting to soak up all things vegan, I recommend:

The Compassionate Road
My Vegan Journal
No Meat Athlete
Rich Roll
The Vegan Strategist
Your Daily Vegan
Food Revolution Network
Peaceful Dumpling
The Beet
Live Kindly

Plant-Based Cookbooks

Investing in a couple of awesome plant-based cookbooks (especially with mouth-watering photos!) really helped me learn the basics of plant-based eating. Of course, that list of plant-based cookbooks has grown from two to about twenty! Here are my favorites because they are whole food based and always so delicious.

Power Plates, Gena Hamshaw

Isa Does It, Isa Chandra Moskowitz

Unbelievably Vegan, Charity Morgan

The First Mess, Laura Wright

Plant Based Cooking Made Easy, Jill Dalton and Jeffrey Dalton

Mississippi Vegan, Timothy Pakron

Afro-Vegan, Bryant Terry

Vegan Richa's Everyday Kitchen, Richa Hingle

Minimalist Baker's Everyday Cooking, Dana Shultz

Homemade Vegan Pantry, Miyoko Shinner

Veganomicon, Isa Chandra Moskowicz and Terry Hope Romero

Recipe Blogs

If you want tried and true delicious vegan recipes, bookmark a handful of recipe blogs that you've either tried and loved or that get rave online reviews. These blogs will come in handy when you're looking to use up ingredients in your fridge or need to make a meal in a pinch. For example, if you purchased kale and used it for one recipe but still have some leftover and are unsure what to do with it, search "kale" in the blog's search bar to find a recipe using kale that piques your interest.

Vegan Richa

The Plant Philosophy

Keepin' It Kind

Healthy Happy Life

Olives for Dinner

Oh Lady Cakes

The First Mess

The Vegan 8

The Full Helping

Nutritiously (includes a meal plan)

Evidence-Based Research Websites

Nutritionfacts.org

Nutritionstudies.org

Foodrevolution.org

Foodempowermentproject.org

Veganrd.com

Veganhealth.org

Pcrm.org

Plantbasedjuniors.com

Vndpg.org

Gssiweb.org

Sportsdietitians.com.au

Books for Inspiration

A Diet for a New America by John Robbins

Becoming Vegan: A Guide to Adopting a Healthy Plant-Based Diet by Brenda Davis and Vesanto Melina

Eat to Live by Dr. Joel Fuhrman

How to Not Die by gene Stone and Dr. Michael gregor

Power Foods for the Brain by Dr. Neal Barnard

The China Study by Dr. T. Colin Campbell and Dr. Thomas M. Campbell

Vegan for Life by Jack Norris and ginny Messina

World Peace Diet: Eating for Spiritual Health and Social Harmony by William Tuttle

Your Body in Balance by Dr. Neal Barnard

Protein Powder Recommendations

Complement

Ora

Truvani

Sprouted Living

Meal Kit Services

Purple Carrot
Daily Harvest
Trifecta Nutrition
Veestro
VegReady
Mamasezz
Foodflo
Hungry Root
Fresh N Lean
The Splendid Spoon

Ethically-Centric Organizations

Movement for Compassionate Living
Vegan Outreach
Mercy for Animals
Farm Sanctuary
Humane Society International
Switch4Good

Works Cited

Why Vegan?

"Iron Consumption Can Increase Risk for Heart Disease, Study Shows." 2014. ScienceDaily. 2014. https://www.sciencedaily.com/releases/2014/04/140423170903. htm.

Chapter 1

"11 Reasons Why Too Much Sugar Is Bad for You." 2018. Healthline. June 3, 2018. https://www.healthline.com/nutrition/sugar-the-worst-ingredient-in-the-diet.

Chapter 2

"Winning Strategy — Address Weight and Energy Intake to Improve Athletes' Performance." n.d. Www.todaysdietitian.com. Accessed May 24, 2023. https://www. todaysdietitian.com/newarchives/111609p14.shtml.

2023. Ncaa.org. 2023. https://www.ncaa.org/sites/default/files/Female%20 Athlete%20Triad.pdf.

August 2016, Tia Ghose 13. n.d. "Here's What Olympians Eat for Each Sport." Livescience.com. https://www.livescience.com/55747-what-olympians-eat.html.

Mifflin, M D, S T St Jeor, L A Hill, B J Scott, S A Daugherty, and Y O Koh. 1990. "A New Predictive Equation for Resting Energy Expenditure in Healthy Individuals." *The American Journal of Clinical Nutrition* 51 (2): 241–47. https://doi.org/10.1093/ ajcn/51.2.241.

Montalcini, Tiziana, Daniele De Bonis, Yvelise Ferro, Ilaria Carè, Elisa Mazza, Francesca Accattato, Marta Greco, et al. 2015. "High Vegetable Fats Intake Is Associated with High Resting Energy Expenditure in Vegetarians." *Nutrients* 7 (7): 5933–47. https://doi.org/10.3390/nu7075259.

Szalay, Jessie. 2015. "What Are Calories?" Live Science. Live Science. November 14, 2015. https://www.livescience.com/52802-what-is-a-calorie.html.

Toth, Michael J., and Eric T. Poehlman. 1994. "Sympathetic Nervous System Activity and Resting Metabolic Rate in Vegetarians." *Metabolism* 43 (5): 621–25. https://doi.org/10.1016/0026-0495(94)90205-4.

Chapter 3

"Appendix 7. Nutritional Goals for Age-Sex Groups Based on Dietary Reference Intakes and Dietary Guidelines Recommendations - 2015-2020 Dietary Guidelines | Health.gov." 2015. Health.gov. 2015. https://health.gov/our-work/food-nutrition/2015-2020-dietary-guidelines/guidelines/appendix-7/.

"Postexercise Recovery — Proper Nutrition Is Key to Refuel, Rehydrate, and Rebuild after Strenuous Workouts." 2013. Todaysdietitian.com. 2013. https://www.todaysdietitian.com/newarchives/110413p18.shtml.

Augustin, L.S.A., C.W.C. Kendall, D.J.A. Jenkins, W.C. Willett, A. Astrup, A.W. Barclay, I. Björck, et al. 2015. "Glycemic Index, Glycemic Load and Glycemic Response: An International Scientific Consensus Summit from the International Carbohydrate Quality Consortium (ICQC)." *Nutrition, Metabolism and Cardiovascular Diseases* 25 (9): 795–815. https://doi.org/10.1016/j.numecd.2015.05.005.

Burdon, Catriona A., Inge Spronk, Hoi Lun Cheng, and Helen T. O'Connor. 2016. "Effect of Glycemic Index of a Pre-Exercise Meal on Endurance Exercise Performance: A Systematic Review and Meta-Analysis." *Sports Medicine* 47 (6): 1087–1101. https://doi.org/10.1007/s40279-016-0632-8.

Burke, L. M., G. R. Collier, and M. Hargreaves. 1993. "Muscle Glycogen Storage after Prolonged Exercise: Effect of the Glycemic Index of Carbohydrate Feedings." *Journal of Applied Physiology* 75 (2): 1019–23. https://doi.org/10.1152/jappl.1993.75.2.1019.

Burke, Louise M., Luc J. C. van Loon, and John A. Hawley. 2017. "Postexercise Muscle Glycogen Resynthesis in Humans." *Journal of Applied Physiology* 122 (5): 1055–67. https://doi.org/10.1152/japplphysiol.00860.2016.

Little, Jonathan P., Philip D. Chilibeck, Dawn Ciona, Scott Forbes, Huw Rees, Albert Vandenberg, and Gordon A. Zello. 2010. "Effect of Low- and High-Glycemic-Index Meals on Metabolism and Performance during High-Intensity, Intermittent Exercise." *International Journal of Sport Nutrition and Exercise Metabolism* 20 (6): 447–56. https://doi.org/10.1123/ijsnem.20.6.447.

Mondazzi, Luca, and Enrico Arcelli. 2009. "Glycemic Index in Sport Nutrition." *Journal of the American College of Nutrition* 28 (sup4): 455S463S. https://doi.org/10.1080/07 315724.2009.10718112.

Murray, Bob, and Christine Rosenbloom. 2018. "Fundamentals of Glycogen Metabolism for Coaches and Athletes." *Nutrition Reviews* 76 (4): 243–59. https://doi. org/10.1093/nutrit/nuy001.

Williams, Clyde, and Ian Rollo. 2015. "Carbohydrate Nutrition and Team Sport Performance." *Sports Medicine* 45 (S1): 13–22. https://doi.org/10.1007/s40279-015-0399-3.

Chapter 4

"Protein and Amino Acids." n.d. VeganHealth.org. Accessed May 24, 2023. https:// veganhealth.org/protein/.

Babault, Nicolas, Christos Païzis, Gaëlle Deley, Laetitia Guérin-Deremaux, Marie-Hélène Saniez, Catherine Lefranc-Millot, and François A Allaert. 2015. "Pea Proteins Oral Supplementation Promotes Muscle Thickness Gains during Resistance Training: A Double-Blind, Randomized, Placebo-Controlled Clinical Trial vs. Whey Protein." *Journal of the International Society of Sports Nutrition* 12 (1): 3. https://doi. org/10.1186/s12970-014-0064-5.

Banaszek, Amy, Jeremy Townsend, David Bender, William Vantrease, Autumn Marshall, and Kent Johnson. 2019. "The Effects of Whey vs. Pea Protein on Physical Adaptations Following 8-Weeks of High-Intensity Functional Training (HIFT): A Pilot Study." *Sports* 7 (1): 12. https://doi.org/10.3390/sports7010012.

Beasley, Jeannette M., A. L. Deierlein, K. B. Morland, E. C. Granieri, and A. Spark. 2016. "Is Meeting the Recommended Dietary Allowance (RDA) for Protein Related to Body Composition among Older Adults?: Results from the Cardiovascular Health of Seniors and Built Environment Study." *The Journal of Nutrition, Health & Aging* 20 (8): 790–96. https://doi.org/10.1007/s12603-015-0707-5.

Dt, Thomas, Erdman Ka, and Burke Lm. 2016. "Position of the Academy of Nutrition and Dietetics, Dietitians of Canada, and the American College of Sports Medicine: Nutrition and Athletic Performance." Journal of the Academy of Nutrition and Dietetics. March 1, 2016. https://pubmed.ncbi.nlm.nih.gov/26920240/.

Jackman, Sarah R., Oliver C. Witard, Andrew Philp, Gareth A. Wallis, Keith Baar, and Kevin D. Tipton. 2017. "Branched-Chain Amino Acid Ingestion Stimulates Muscle Myofibrillar Protein Synthesis Following Resistance Exercise in Humans." *Frontiers in Physiology* 8 (June). https://doi.org/10.3389/fphys.2017.00390.

Jäger, Ralf, Chad M. Kerksick, Bill I. Campbell, Paul J. Cribb, Shawn D. Wells, Tim M. Skwiat, Martin Purpura, et al. 2017. "International Society of Sports Nutrition Position Stand: Protein and Exercise." *Journal of the International Society of Sports Nutrition* 14 (1). https://doi.org/10.1186/s12970-017-0177-8.

Kerksick, Chad M., Shawn Arent, Brad J. Schoenfeld, Jeffrey R. Stout, Bill Campbell, Colin D. Wilborn, Lem Taylor, et al. 2017. "International Society of Sports Nutrition Position Stand: Nutrient Timing." *Journal of the International Society of Sports Nutrition* 14 (1). https://doi.org/10.1186/s12970-017-0189-4.

Lemon, Peter & Yarasheski, Kevin & Dolny, Dennis. 1984. The Importance of Protein for Athletes. Sports medicine (Auckland, N.Z.). 1. 474-84. 10.2165/00007256-198401060-00006.

McDonald, Cameron Keith, Mikkel Z. Ankarfeldt, Sandra Capra, Judy Bauer, Kyle Raymond, and Berit Lilienthal Heitmann. 2016. "Lean Body Mass Change over 6 Years Is Associated with Dietary Leucine Intake in an Older Danish Population." *British Journal of Nutrition* 115 (9): 1556–62. https://doi.org/10.1017/s0007114516000611.

Phillips, Stuart M., and Luc J.C. Van Loon. 2011. "Dietary Protein for Athletes: From Requirements to Optimum Adaptation." *Journal of Sports Sciences* 29 (sup1): S29–38. https://doi.org/10.1080/02640414.2011.619204.

Stellingwerff, Trent, Ronald J. Maughan, and Louise M. Burke. 2011. "Nutrition for Power Sports: Middle-Distance Running, Track Cycling, Rowing, Canoeing/Kayaking, and Swimming." *Journal of Sports Sciences* 29 (sup1): S79–89. https://doi.org/10.1080/02640414.2011.589469.

Tipton, Kevin D, and Robert R Wolfe. 2004. "Protein and Amino Acids for Athletes." *Journal of Sports Sciences* 22 (1): 65–79. https://doi.org/10.1080/0264041031000140554.

Chapter 5

"Vegetarian's Challenge — Optimizing Essential Fatty Acid Status." n.d. Www.todaysdietitian.com. Accessed May 24, 2023. https://www.todaysdietitian.com/newarchives/020810p22.shtml.

Brennan, Sarah F., Jayne V. Woodside, Paula M. Lunny, Chris R. Cardwell, and Marie M. Cantwell. 2015. "Dietary Fat and Breast Cancer Mortality: A Systematic Review and Meta-Analysis." *Critical Reviews in Food Science and Nutrition* 57 (10): 1999–2008. https://doi.org/10.1080/10408398.2012.724481.

Costantini, Lara, Romina Molinari, Barbara Farinon, and Nicolò Merendino. 2017. "Impact of Omega-3 Fatty Acids on the Gut Microbiota." *International Journal of Molecular Sciences* 18 (12): 2645. https://doi.org/10.3390/ijms18122645.

Di Sebastiano, Katie M., and Marina Mourtzakis. 2014. "The Role of Dietary Fat throughout the Prostate Cancer Trajectory." *Nutrients* 6 (12): 6095–6109. https://doi.org/10.3390/nu6126095.

Fritsche, Kevin L. 2015. "The Science of Fatty Acids and Inflammation123." *Advances in Nutrition* 6 (3): 293S301S. https://doi.org/10.3945/an.114.006940.

González, Frank, Robert V Considine, Ola A Abdelhadi, and Anthony J Acton. 2018. "Saturated Fat Ingestion Promotes Lipopolysaccharide-Mediated Inflammation and Insulin Resistance in Polycystic Ovary Syndrome." *The Journal of Clinical Endocrinology & Metabolism* 104 (3): 934–46. https://doi.org/10.1210/jc.2018-01143.

Harvard Health Publishing. 2019. "Do Omega-3s Protect Your Thinking Skills? - Harvard Health." Harvard Health. Harvard Health. May 3, 2019. https://www.health.harvard.edu/staying-healthy/do-omega-3s-protect-your-thinking-skills.

Harvard Health Publishing. 2019. "The Truth about Fats: The Good, the Bad, and the In-Between." Harvard Health. Harvard Health. December 11, 2019. https://www.health.harvard.edu/staying-healthy/the-truth-about-fats-bad-and-good.

Herbert, Diana, Sandra Franz, Yulia Popkova, Ulf Anderegg, Jürgen Schiller, Katharina Schwede, Axel Lorz, Jan C. Simon, and Anja Saalbach. 2018. "High-Fat Diet Exacerbates Early Psoriatic Skin Inflammation Independent of Obesity: Saturated Fatty Acids as Key Players." *Journal of Investigative Dermatology* 138 (9): 1999–2009. https://doi.org/10.1016/j.jid.2018.03.1522.

Hooper L, Martin N, Abdelhamid A, Davey Smith G. Reduction in saturated fat intake for cardiovascular disease. Cochrane Database of Systematic Reviews 2015, Issue 6. Art. No.: CD011737. DOI: 10.1002/14651858.CD011737.

Publishing, Harvard Health. 2019. "No Need to Avoid Healthy Omega-6 Fats." Harvard Health. August 20, 2019. https://www.health.harvard.edu/newsletter_article/no-need-to-avoid-healthy-omega-6-fats.

Swanson, Danielle, Robert Block, and Shaker A. Mousa. 2012. "Omega-3 Fatty Acids EPA and DHA: Health Benefits throughout Life." *Advances in Nutrition* 3 (1): 1–7. https://doi.org/10.3945/an.111.000893.

Wolters, Maike, Jenny Ahrens, Marina Romaní-Pérez, Claire Watkins, Yolanda Sanz, Alfonso Benítez-Páez, Catherine Stanton, and Kathrin Günther. 2019. "Dietary Fat, the Gut Microbiota, and Metabolic Health – a Systematic Review Conducted within the MyNewGut Project." *Clinical Nutrition* 38 (6): 2504–20. https://doi.org/10.1016/j.clnu.2018.12.024.

Chapter 6

"The Microbiota in Exercise Immunology." 2015. http://eir-isei.de/2015/eir-2015-070-article.pdf.

Barton, Wiley, Nicholas C Penney, Owen Cronin, Isabel Garcia-Perez, Michael G Molloy, Elaine Holmes, Fergus Shanahan, Paul D Cotter, and Orla O'Sullivan. 2017. "The Microbiome of Professional Athletes Differs from that of More Sedentary Subjects in Composition and Particularly at the Functional Metabolic Level." *Gut* 67 (4): gutjnl-2016-313627. https://doi.org/10.1136/gutjnl-2016-313627.

Jang, Lae-Guen, Geunhoon Choi, Sung-Woo Kim, Byung-Yong Kim, Sunghee Lee, and Hyon Park. 2019. "The Combination of Sport and Sport-Specific Diet Is Associated with Characteristics of Gut Microbiota: An Observational Study." *Journal of the International Society of Sports Nutrition* 16 (1). https://doi.org/10.1186/s12970-019-0290-y.

Mach, Núria, and Dolors Fuster-Botella. 2017. "Endurance Exercise and Gut Microbiota: A Review." *Journal of Sport and Health Science* 6 (2): 179–97. https://doi.org/10.1016/j.jshs.2016.05.001.

Petersen, Lauren M., Eddy J. Bautista, Hoan Nguyen, Blake M. Hanson, Lei Chen, Sai H. Lek, Erica Sodergren, and George M. Weinstock. 2017. "Community Characteristics of the Gut Microbiomes of Competitive Cyclists." *Microbiome* 5 (1). https://doi.org/10.1186/s40168-017-0320-4.

Scheiman, Jonathan, Jacob M. Luber, Theodore A. Chavkin, Tara MacDonald, Angela Tung, Loc-Duyen Pham, Marsha C. Wibowo, et al. 2019. "Meta-Omics Analysis of Elite Athletes Identifies a Performance-Enhancing Microbe That Functions via Lactate Metabolism." *Nature Medicine* 25 (7): 1104–9. https://doi.org/10.1038/s41591-019-0485-4.

Chapter 7

Belval, Luke N., Yuri Hosokawa, Douglas J. Casa, William M. Adams, Lawrence E. Armstrong, Lindsay B. Baker, Louise Burke, et al. 2019. "Practical Hydration Solutions for Sports." *Nutrients* 11 (7): 1550. https://doi.org/10.3390/nu11071550.

Cheuvront, Samuel N., and Robert W. Kenefick. 2016. "Am I Drinking Enough? Yes, No, and Maybe." *Journal of the American College of Nutrition* 35 (2): 185–92. https://doi.org/10.1080/07315724.2015.1067872.

Sports Dietitians Australia. 2015. "Fluids in Sport - Sports Dietitians Australia (SDA)." Sports Dietitians Australia (SDA). 2015. https://www.sportsdietitians.com.au/factsheets/fuelling-recovery/fluids-in-sport/.

Chapter 8

Bolland, M. J., A. Avenell, J. A. Baron, A. Grey, G. S. MacLennan, G. D. Gamble, and I. R. Reid. 2010. "Effect of Calcium Supplements on Risk of Myocardial Infarction and Cardiovascular Events: Meta-Analysis." *BMJ* 341 (jul29 1): c3691–91. https://doi.org/10.1136/bmj.c3691.

Mayo Clinic. 2018. "Are You Getting Enough Calcium?" Mayo Clinic. October 3, 2018. https://www.mayoclinic.org/healthy-lifestyle/nutrition-and-healthy-eating/in-depth/calcium-supplements/art-20047097.

Rogerson, David. 2017. "Vegan Diets: Practical Advice for Athletes and Exercisers." *Journal of the International Society of Sports Nutrition* 14 (1). https://doi.org/10.1186/s12970-017-0192-9.

Sale, Craig, and Kirsty Jayne Elliott-Sale. 2019. "Nutrition and Athlete Bone Health." *Sports Medicine* 49 (2). https://doi.org/10.1007/s40279-019-01161-2.

Tang, Anne, Karen Walker Phd, Gisela Wilcox, Boyd Strauss, John Ashton, and Lily Stojanovska. 2010. "Calcium Absorption in Australian Osteopenic Post-Menopausal Women: An Acute Comparative Study of Fortified Soymilk to Cows' Milk." *Asia Pac J Clin Nutr* 19 (2): 243–49. http://apjcn.nhri.org.tw/server/APJCN/19/2/243.pdf.

Chapter 9

Lombardi, Giovanni, Jacopo Antonino Vitale, Sergio Logoluso, Giovanni Logoluso, Nino Cocco, Giulio Cocco, Antonino Cocco, and Giuseppe Banfi. 2017. "Circannual Rhythm of Plasmatic Vitamin D Levels and the Association with Markers of Psychophysical Stress in a Cohort of Italian Professional Soccer Players." *Chronobiology International* 34 (4): 471–79. https://doi.org/10.1080/07420528.2017.1297820.

Pludowski, Pawel, Michael F. Holick, William B. Grant, Jerzy Konstantynowicz, Mario R. Mascarenhas, Afrozul Haq, Vladyslav Povoroznyuk, et al. 2018. "Vitamin D Supplementation Guidelines." *The Journal of Steroid Biochemistry and Molecular Biology* 175 (January): 125–35. https://doi.org/10.1016/j.jsbmb.2017.01.021.

Rogerson, David. 2017. "Vegan Diets: Practical Advice for Athletes and Exercisers." *Journal of the International Society of Sports Nutrition* 14 (1). https://doi.org/10.1186/s12970-017-0192-9.

Romagnoli, Elisabetta, Maria Lucia Mascia, Cristiana Cipriani, Valeria Fassino, Franco Mazzei, Emilio D'Erasmo, Vincenzo Carnevale, Alfredo Scillitani, and Salvatore Minisola. 2008. "Short and Long-Term Variations in Serum Calciotropic Hormones after a Single Very Large Dose of Ergocalciferol (Vitamin D2) or Cholecalciferol (Vitamin D3) in the Elderly." *The Journal of Clinical Endocrinology and Metabolism* 93 (8): 3015–20. https://doi.org/10.1210/jc.2008-0350.

Sikora-Klak, Jakub, Steven J Narvy, Justin Yang, Eric Makhni, F Daniel Kharrazi, and Nima Mehran. 2018. "The Effect of Abnormal Vitamin D Levels in Athletes." *The Permanente Journal* 22 (July). https://doi.org/10.7812/TPP/17-216.

Chapter 10

Alaunyte, Ieva, Valentina Stojceska, and Andrew Plunkett. 2015. "Iron and the Female Athlete: A Review of Dietary Treatment Methods for Improving Iron Status and Exercise Performance." *Journal of the International Society of Sports Nutrition* 12 (1). https://doi.org/10.1186/s12970-015-0099-2.

Burden, Richard J., Katie Morton, Toby Richards, Gregory P. Whyte, and Charles R. Pedlar. 2015. "Is Iron Treatment Beneficial In, Iron-Deficient but Non-Anaemic (IDNA) Endurance Athletes? A Systematic Review and Meta-Analysis." *British Journal of Sports Medicine* 49 (21): 1389–97. https://doi.org/10.1136/bjsports-2014-093624.

Institute of Medicine (US) Panel on Micronutrients. 2014. "Iron." Nih.gov. National Academies Press (US). 2014. https://www.ncbi.nlm.nih.gov/books/NBK222309/.

Lönnerdal, Bo, Annika Bryant, Xiaofeng Liu, and Elizabeth C Theil. 2006. "Iron Absorption from Soybean Ferritin in Nonanemic Women." *The American Journal of Clinical Nutrition* 83 (1): 103–7. https://doi.org/10.1093/ajcn/83.1.103.

Warner, Matthew J, and Muhammad T Kamran. 2022. "Iron Deficiency Anemia." Nih.gov. StatPearls Publishing. August 8, 2022. https://www.ncbi.nlm.nih.gov/books/NBK448065/.

Zimmermann, Michael B, and Richard F Hurrell. 2007. "Nutritional Iron Deficiency." *The Lancet* 370 (9586): 511–20. https://doi.org/10.1016/s0140-6736(07)61235-5.

Chapter 11

"Vitamin B12." 2014. Linus Pauling Institute. April 22, 2014. https://lpi.oregonstate.edu/mic/vitamins/vitamin-B12.

Adams, J F, Sheila A Ross, L Mervyn, K Boddy, and Priscilla C King. 1971. "Absorption of Cyanocobalamin, Coenzyme B_{12}, Methylcobalamin, and Hydroxocobalamin at Different Dose Levels." *Scandinavian Journal of Gastroenterology* 6 (3): 249–52. https://doi.org/10.3109/00365527109180702.

Dahele, Anna, and Subrata Ghosh. 2001. "Vitamin B12 Deficiency in Untreated Celiac Disease." *The American Journal of Gastroenterology* 96 (3): 745–50. https://doi.org/10.1111/j.1572-0241.2001.03616.x.

Habte, Kifle, Abdulaziz Adish, Dilnesaw Zerfu, Aweke Kebede, Tibebu Moges, Biniyam Tesfaye, Feyissa Challa, and Kaleab Baye. 2015. "Iron, Folate and Vitamin B12 Status of Ethiopian Professional Runners." *Nutrition & Metabolism* 12 (1). https://doi.org/10.1186/s12986-015-0056-8.

Marcil, Valérie, Emile Levy, Devendra Amre, Alain Bitton, Ana Maria Guilhon de Araújo Sant'Anna, Andrew Szilagy, Daniel Sinnett, and Ernest G Seidman. 2019. "A Cross-Sectional Study on Malnutrition in Inflammatory Bowel Disease: Is There a Difference Based on Pediatric or Adult Age Grouping?" *Inflammatory Bowel Diseases* 25 (8): 1428–41. https://doi.org/10.1093/ibd/izy403.

Paul, Cristiana, and David M. Brady. 2017. "Comparative Bioavailability and Utilization of Particular Forms of B12 Supplements with Potential to Mitigate B12-Related Genetic Polymorphisms." *Integrative Medicine (Encinitas, Calif.)* 16 (1): 42–49. https://pubmed.ncbi.nlm.nih.gov/28223907.

Chapter 12

"Iodine Deficiency." n.d. American Thyroid Association. Accessed May 24, 2023. http://www.thyroid.org/iodine-deficiency/.

Institute of Medicine (US) Panel on Micronutrients. 2012. "Iodine." Nih.gov. National Academies Press (US). 2012. https://www.ncbi.nlm.nih.gov/books/NBK222323/.

Institute of Medicine (US) Panel on Micronutrients. 2012. "Iodine." Nih.gov. National Academies Press (US). 2012. https://www.ncbi.nlm.nih.gov/books/NBK222323/.

Chapter 13

DiNicolantonio, James J, James H O'Keefe, and William Wilson. 2018. "Subclinical Magnesium Deficiency: A Principal Driver of Cardiovascular Disease and a Public Health Crisis." *Open Heart* 5 (1): e000668. https://doi.org/10.1136/openhrt-2017-000668.

DiNicolantonio, James J, James H O'Keefe, and William Wilson. 2018. "Subclinical Magnesium Deficiency: A Principal Driver of Cardiovascular Disease and a Public Health Crisis." *Open Heart* 5 (1): e000668. https://doi.org/10.1136/openhrt-2017-000668.

Kass, Lindsy S, and Filipe Poeira. 2015. "The Effect of Acute vs Chronic Magnesium Supplementation on Exercise and Recovery on Resistance Exercise, Blood Pressure and Total Peripheral Resistance on Normotensive Adults." *Journal of the International Society of Sports Nutrition* 12 (1). https://doi.org/10.1186/s12970-015-0081-z.

Nielsen, F. H., and H. C. Lukaski. 2006. "Update on the Relationship between Magnesium and Exercise." *Magnesium Research* 19 (3): 180–89. https://pubmed.ncbi.nlm.nih.gov/17172008/.

Chapter 15

Baltaci, Abdulkerim Kasim, Rasim Mogulkoc, Mustafa Akil, and Mursel Bicer. 2016. "Review - Selenium - Its Metabolism and Relation to Exercise." *Pakistan Journal of Pharmaceutical Sciences* 29 (5): 1719–25. https://pubmed.ncbi.nlm.nih.gov/27731835/.

Bolling, Bradley W., C.-Y. Oliver Chen, Diane L. McKay, and Jeffrey B. Blumberg. 2011. "Tree Nut Phytochemicals: Composition, Antioxidant Capacity, Bioactivity, Impact Factors. A Systematic Review of Almonds, Brazils, Cashews, Hazelnuts, Macadamias, Pecans, Pine Nuts, Pistachios and Walnuts." *Nutrition Research Reviews* 24 (2): 244–75. https://doi.org/10.1017/s095442241100014x.

Del Gobbo, Liana C, Michael C Falk, Robin Feldman, Kara Lewis, and Dariush Mozaffarian. 2015. "Effects of Tree Nuts on Blood Lipids, Apolipoproteins, and

Blood Pressure: Systematic Review, Meta-Analysis, and Dose-Response of 61 Controlled Intervention Trials." *The American Journal of Clinical Nutrition* 102 (6): 1347–56. https://doi.org/10.3945/ajcn.115.110965.

Fernández-Lázaro, Diego, Cesar I. Fernandez-Lazaro, Juan Mielgo-Ayuso, Lourdes Jiménez Navascués, Alfredo Córdova Martínez, and Jesús Seco-Calvo. 2020. "The Role of Selenium Mineral Trace Element in Exercise: Antioxidant Defense System, Muscle Performance, Hormone Response, and Athletic Performance. A Systematic Review." *Nutrients* 12 (6): 1790. https://doi.org/10.3390/nu12061790.

Gill, Harsharn, and Glen Walker. 2008. "Selenium, Immune Function and Resistance to Viral Infections." *Nutrition & Dietetics* 65 (June): S41–47. https://doi.org/10.1111/j.1747-0080.2008.00260.x.

Maynar, Marcos, Diego Muñoz, Javier Alves, Gema Barrientos, Francisco Javier Grijota, María Concepción Robles, and Francisco Llerena. 2018. "Influence of an Acute Exercise until Exhaustion on Serum and Urinary Concentrations of Molybdenum, Selenium, and Zinc in Athletes." *Biological Trace Element Research* 186 (2): 361–69. https://doi.org/10.1007/s12011-018-1327-9.

Wu, Qian, Margaret P. Rayman, Hongjun Lv, Lutz Schomburg, Bo Cui, Chuqi Gao, Pu Chen, et al. 2015. "Low Population Selenium Status Is Associated with Increased Prevalence of Thyroid Disease." *The Journal of Clinical Endocrinology & Metabolism* 100 (11): 4037–47. https://doi.org/10.1210/jc.2015-2222.

Chapter 16

Bielohuby, Maximilian, Maiko Matsuura, Nadja Herbach, Ellen Kienzle, Marc Slawik, Andreas Hoeflich, and Martin Bidlingmaier. 2009. "Short-Term Exposure to Low-Carbohydrate, High-Fat Diets Induces Low Bone Mineral Density and Reduces Bone Formation in Rats." *Journal of Bone and Mineral Research* 25 (2): 275–84. https://doi.org/10.1359/jbmr.090813.

Conaway, H. Herschel, Petra Henning, and Ulf H. Lerner. 2013. "Vitamin a Metabolism, Action, and Role in Skeletal Homeostasis." *Endocrine Reviews* 34 (6): 766–97. https://doi.org/10.1210/er.2012-1071.

Haakonssen, Eric C et al. "The effects of a calcium-rich pre-exercise meal on biomarkers of calcium homeostasis in competitive female cyclists: a randomised crossover trial." PloS one vol. 10,5 e0123302. 13 May. 2015, doi:10.1371/journal.pone.0123302

National Institutes of Health. 2017. "Office of Dietary Supplements - Vitamin K." Nih. gov. 2017. https://ods.od.nih.gov/factsheets/vitaminK-HealthProfessional/.

Robbins, Ocean. 2020. "How to Prevent Osteoporosis and Promote Bone Health with Food." Food Revolution Network. July 17, 2020. https://foodrevolution.org/blog/how-to-prevent-osteoporosis.

Sale, Craig, and Kirsty Jayne Elliott-Sale. 2019. "Nutrition and Athlete Bone Health." *Sports Medicine* 49 (2). https://doi.org/10.1007/s40279-019-01161-2.

Sale, Craig, and Kirsty Jayne Elliott-Sale. 2019. "Nutrition and Athlete Bone Health." *Sports Medicine* 49 (2). https://doi.org/10.1007/s40279-019-01161-2.

Tong, Tammy Y. N., Paul N. Appleby, Miranda E. G. Armstrong, Georgina K. Fensom, Anika Knuppel, Keren Papier, Aurora Perez-Cornago, Ruth C. Travis, and Timothy J. Key. 2020. "Vegetarian and Vegan Diets and Risks of Total and Site-Specific Fractures: Results from the Prospective EPIC-Oxford Study." *BMC Medicine* 18 (1). https://doi.org/10.1186/s12916-020-01815-3.

Chapter 17

Bowtell, Joanna, and Vincent Kelly. 2019. "Fruit-Derived Polyphenol Supplementation for Athlete Recovery and Performance." *Sports Medicine* 49 (S1): 3–23. https://doi.org/10.1007/s40279-018-0998-x.

Cheung, Karoline, Patria A Hume, and Linda Maxwell. 2003. "Delayed Onset Muscle Soreness." *Sports Medicine* 33 (2): 145–64. https://doi.org/10.2165/00007256-200333020-00005.

Merghani, Ahmed, Viviana Maestrini, Stefania Rosmini, Andrew T. Cox, Harshil Dhutia, Rachel Bastiaenan, Sarojini David, et al. 2017. "Prevalence of Subclinical Coronary Artery Disease in Masters Endurance Athletes with a Low Atherosclerotic Risk Profile." *Circulation* 136 (2): 126–37. https://doi.org/10.1161/circulationaha.116.026964.

Pahwa, Roma, Amandeep Goyal, Pankaj Bansal, and Ishwarlal Jialal. 2020. "Chronic Inflammation." PubMed. Treasure Island (FL): StatPearls Publishing. 2020. https://www.ncbi.nlm.nih.gov/books/NBK493173.

Schwartz, Robert S, Stacia Merkel Kraus, Jonathan G Schwartz, Kelly K Wickstrom, Gretchen Peichel, Ross F Garberich, John R Lesser, et al. 2014. "Increased Coronary Artery Plaque Volume among Male Marathon Runners." *Missouri Medicine* 111 (2): 89–94. https://www.ncbi.nlm.nih.gov/pmc/articles/PMC6179497.

Chapter 18

"What You Eat Can Influence How You Sleep: Daily Intake of Fiber, Saturated Fat and Sugar May Impact Sleep Quality." n.d. ScienceDaily. https://www.sciencedaily.com/releases/2016/01/160114213443.htm.

CDC. 2017. "CDC - Data and Statistics - Sleep and Sleep Disorders." Centers for Disease Control and Prevention. 2017. https://www.cdc.gov/sleep/data_statistics.html.

CDC. 2017. "CDC - Data and Statistics - Sleep and Sleep Disorders." Centers for Disease Control and Prevention. 2017. https://www.cdc.gov/sleep/data_statistics.html.

Hart, Chantelle N., Mary A. Carskadon, Kathryn E. Demos, Eliza Van Reen, Katherine M. Sharkey, Hollie A. Raynor, Robert V. Considine, Richard N. Jones, and Rena R. Wing. 2014. "Acute Changes in Sleep Duration on Eating Behaviors and Appetite-Regulating Hormones in Overweight/Obese Adults." *Behavioral Sleep Medicine* 13 (5): 424–36. https://doi.org/10.1080/15402002.2014.940105.

Krause, Adam J., Eti Ben Simon, Bryce A. Mander, Stephanie M. Greer, Jared M. Saletin, Andrea N. Goldstein-Piekarski, and Matthew P. Walker. 2017. "The Sleep-Deprived Human Brain." *Nature Reviews Neuroscience* 18 (7): 404–18. https://doi.org/10.1038/nrn.2017.55.

Mazzotti Diego Robles, Guindalini Camila, Moraes Walter André dos Santos, Andersen Monica Levy, Cendoroglo Maysa Seabra, Ramos Luiz Roberto, Tufik Sergio. "Human longevity is associated with regular sleep patterns, maintenance of slow wave sleep, and favorable lipid profile." Frontiers in Aging Neuroscience Vol. 6. 2014.

Sharma, Sunil, and Mani Kavuru. 2010. "Sleep and Metabolism: An Overview." *International Journal of Endocrinology* 2010 (August): 1–12. https://doi.org/10.1155/2010/270832.

St-Onge, Marie-Pierre, Allison Crawford, and Brooke Aggarwal. 2018. "Plant-Based Diets: Reducing Cardiovascular Risk by Improving Sleep Quality?" *Current Sleep Medicine Reports* 4 (1): 74–78. https://www.ncbi.nlm.nih.gov/pmc/articles/PMC5999325.

St-Onge, Marie-Pierre, Allison Crawford, and Brooke Aggarwal. 2018. "Plant-Based Diets: Reducing Cardiovascular Risk by Improving Sleep Quality?" *Current Sleep Medicine Reports* 4 (1): 74–78. https://www.ncbi.nlm.nih.gov/pmc/articles/PMC5999325/.

St-Onge, Marie-Pierre, Allison Crawford, and Brooke Aggarwal. 2018. "Plant-Based Diets: Reducing Cardiovascular Risk by Improving Sleep Quality?" *Current Sleep Medicine Reports* 4 (1): 74–78. https://www.ncbi.nlm.nih.gov/pmc/articles/PMC5999325/.

Chapter 19

"The Public Health and Safety Organization." n.d. NSF International. https://www.nsf.org.

Aaserud, R., P. Gramvik, S. R. Olsen, and J. Jensen. 1998. "Creatine Supplementation Delays Onset of Fatigue during Repeated Bouts of Sprint Running." *Scandinavian Journal of Medicine & Science in Sports* 8 (5): 247–51. https://doi.org/10.1111/j.1600-0838.1998.tb00478.x.

Alehagen, Urban, Jan Aaseth, Jan Alexander, and Peter Johansson. 2018. "Still Reduced Cardiovascular Mortality 12 Years after Supplementation with Selenium and Coenzyme Q10 for Four Years: A Validation of Previous 10-Year Follow-up Results of a Prospective Randomized Double-Blind Placebo-Controlled Trial in Elderly." Edited by Doan TM Ngo. *PLOS ONE* 13 (4): e0193120. https://doi.org/10.1371/journal.pone.0193120.

Brazier, Yvette. 2017. "What Causes Fatigue, and How Can I Treat It?" Medical News Today. Medical News Today. August 15, 2017. https://www.medicalnewstoday.com/articles/248002.php.

Del Pozo-Cruz, Jesús, Elisabet Rodríguez-Bies, Manuel Ballesteros-Simarro, Ignacio Navas-Enamorado, Bui Thanh Tung, Plácido Navas, and Guillermo López-Lluch. 2014. "Physical Activity Affects Plasma Coenzyme Q10 Levels Differently in Young and Old Humans." *Biogerontology* 15 (2): 199–211. https://doi.org/10.1007/s10522-013-9491-y.

Dodd, F. L., D. O. Kennedy, L. M. Riby, and C. F. Haskell-Ramsay. 2015. "A Double-Blind, Placebo-Controlled Study Evaluating the Effects of Caffeine and L-Theanine Both Alone and in Combination on Cerebral Blood Flow, Cognition and Mood." *Psychopharmacology* 232 (14): 2563–76. https://doi.org/10.1007/s00213-015-3895-0.

Evans, Mark, Peter Tierney, Nicola Gray, Greg Hawe, Maria Macken, and Brendan Egan. 2018. "Acute Ingestion of Caffeinated Chewing Gum Improves Repeated Sprint Performance of Team Sport Athletes with Low Habitual Caffeine Consumption." *International Journal of Sport Nutrition and Exercise Metabolism* 28 (3): 221–27. https://doi.org/10.1123/ijsnem.2017-0217.

Gao, Ruirui, and Philip D. Chilibeck. 2020. "Effect of Tart Cherry Concentrate on Endurance Exercise Performance: A Meta-Analysis." *Journal of the American College of Nutrition*, January, 1–8. https://doi.org/10.1080/07315724.2020.1713246.

Graham, T. E., E. Hibbert, and P. Sathasivam. 1998. "Metabolic and Exercise Endurance Effects of Coffee and Caffeine Ingestion." *Journal of Applied Physiology* 85 (3): 883–89. https://doi.org/10.1152/jappl.1998.85.3.883. https://insights.ovid.com/pubmed?pmid=20019636

Kelly, Simon P., Manuel Gomez-Ramirez, Jennifer L. Montesi, and John J. Foxe. 2008. "L-Theanine and Caffeine in Combination Affect Human Cognition as Evidenced by Oscillatory Alpha-Band Activity and Attention Task Performance." *The Journal of Nutrition* 138 (8): 1572S1577S. https://doi.org/10.1093/jn/138.8.1572s.

Levers, Kyle, Ryan Dalton, Elfego Galvan, Abigail O'Connor, Chelsea Goodenough, Sunday Simbo, Susanne U. Mertens-Talcott, et al. 2016. "Effects of Powdered Montmorency Tart Cherry Supplementation on Acute Endurance Exercise Performance in Aerobically Trained Individuals." *Journal of the International Society of Sports Nutrition* 13 (1). https://doi.org/10.1186/s12970-016-0133-z.

Levers, Kyle, Ryan Dalton, Elfego Galvan, Chelsea Goodenough, Abigail O'Connor, Sunday Simbo, Nicholas Barringer, et al. 2015. "Effects of Powdered Montmorency Tart Cherry Supplementation on an Acute Bout of Intense Lower Body Strength Exercise in Resistance Trained Males." *Journal of the International Society of Sports Nutrition* 12 (1). https://doi.org/10.1186/s12970-015-0102-y.

Machado, Álvaro S., Willian da Silva, Mauren A. Souza, and Felipe P. Carpes. 2018. "Green Tea Extract Preserves Neuromuscular Activation and Muscle Damage Markers in Athletes under Cumulative Fatigue." *Frontiers in Physiology* 9: 1137. https://doi.org/10.3389/fphys.2018.01137.

Newman, Tim. 2017. "Central Nervous System: Structure, Function, and Diseases." Medical News Today. December 22, 2017. https://www.medicalnewstoday.com/articles/307076.php.

Spindler, Meredith, M Flint Beal, and Claire Henchcliffe. 2009. "Coenzyme Q10 Effects in Neurodegenerative Disease." *Neuropsychiatric Disease and Treatment* 5: 597–610. https://www.ncbi.nlm.nih.gov/pmc/articles/PMC2785862/.

U.S. Food and Drug Administration. 2022. "FDA 101: Dietary Supplements." U.S. Food and Drug Administration. June 2, 2022. https://www.fda.gov/consumers/consumer-updates/fda-101-dietary-supplements.

Vitale, Kenneth C., Shawn Hueglin, and Elizabeth Broad. 2017. "Tart Cherry Juice in Athletes." *Current Sports Medicine Reports* 16 (4): 230–39. https://doi.org/10.1249/jsr.0000000000000385.